Be the Lighthouse

A Journey through Kundalini Yoga and Bound Lotus

To Niwan and Harimander, Thank you again for letting me stay with you! Hope to see you at Solstice soon. Sat nam, Abhai Sukai Singh

My experiences with Kundalini Yoga as Taught by Yogi Bhajan® By Steve Coffing

First published by Dog Ear Publishing
4010 W. 86th Street, Ste H
Indianapolis, IN 46268
www.dogearpublishing.net

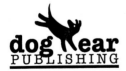

ISBN: 1-59858-188-0
Library of Congress Control Number: 2006930892

This book is printed on acid-free paper.

Printed in the United States of America

Disclaimer

The information contained in this book comes from my impressions and interpretations of what I've experienced while practicing Kundalini Yoga and White Tantric Yoga.

Nothing in this book should be construed as medical advice. While Bound Lotus and the meditations and yoga sets mentioned in this book have benefited many, this book makes no claim to diagnose, treat, cure or prevent any disease, illness, or other condition.

Always check with your personal physician or licensed health care practitioner before making any significant modifications to your lifestyle, to insure that the lifestyle changes, are appropriate for your personal health condition and consistent with any medication you may be taking.

It is recommended that you receive instruction from a KRI certified Kundalini Yoga teacher before attempting any of the postures, kriyas, or meditations mentioned in this book.

For Catherine

Foreword

I had the pleasure of meeting Steve when he was taking Kundalini Yoga Teacher Training in New Mexico in the summer of 2005, and we struck up a friendship afterwards on email. He would often include something he had just written, usually on the subject of his practice of Bound Lotus, so I had a sneak preview of his new book in this way.

Later he was kind enough to take on the seva of typing Yogi Bhajan's lectures from old issues of *Beads of Truth* and *Keeping Up Connections* for the Yogi Bhajan Lecture Library on KRI's website. It seemed he could not get enough of the Teachings, in one form or another! Steve had received his spiritual name by this time—Akal Sahai Singh—which reflects his nature as a true yogi, disciplined and pure. You are sure to find his experience, his dedication and his heartfelt perspective on his personal transformation, refreshing and encouraging to your own practice. Read it all in one sitting, or read a page a day—you are sure to enjoy it either way!

Nam Kaur Khalsa

KRI Executive Director, Yogi Bhajan's Teachings

Introduction

*T*his all began, what seems like so many lifetimes ago, before I let go and made the decision to be the lighthouse....

During my Kundalini Yoga teacher training, we were shown the Yogi Bhajan tribute video, *You Are The Lighthouse*. To say that it changed my life is a supreme understatement. My entire life crystallized when he said, "Be the lighthouse," and that's what I've dedicated my life to doing, to spreading the light.

That's where this book came from, and the title of course. I wrote the first page of what begins on page 5 of this book right afterwards and read it to my class.

I didn't really think much about it, it just was. It received glowing praise and I was encouraged to share my gift. That's what this book is all about. It just comes to me and I write it down.

Much of it is my experiences practicing Kundalini Yoga and Bound Lotus in particular, today was day 183 and I plan never to stop. There's also a lot of things about life in general, all things that come to me along the path of life.

Thank you Catherine for all of your encouragement, receptivity and enthusiasm, this book's for you.

Happy reading, may you find within these pages the inspiration to carry you through all your days and nights.

Bless you, Sat Nam
Steve Coffing
(Akal Sahai Singh)

White Tantric Yoga
through an eagle's eyes

*F*ascinated with eagles as I've always been, I've often wondered what it would be like to soar high above the all. Today I caught a glimpse of what it must be like.

Peering into the eyes of my friend, my partner, I saw her soul across all time and space.

We truly are eternal beings, existing here and there, wherever there is something for us to learn, some magical happening for us to experience.

Perched in the highest tree, waiting for the perfect updraft....
There!

Up into the air with a mighty leap, wings spread wide, soaring high above the all… Free at last, free at last....

For Margaret

*B*lessed be the words, "Dos minutos."

The arms do not go down, no discussion.

But they want to go down, *"Put them down, the pain will go away."*

"No!" The little eagle shouts, "You're trying to trick me into giving up on myself."

Half an hour later, the arms burn, crying for release. Again the eagle shouts, "No! The arms stay up!"

Another half an hour later, the arms cease to exist. All the eagle sees are the eyes of his partner, for all else has long since faded into a white blur.

Then come the magic words, "Dos minutos."

Two minutes later, our eagle puts it's arms down, having prevailed....

Leaving the Nest

*T*he eagle found himself, in the mountains high above the desert.

No, he wasn't lost, he had found his inner being, his spirit, his purpose for being.

He had come to help, in any way that he could. It was time to leave the nest and get on with it.

Along the way he met the Golden Lady, and even an angel who gave him the courage to take that leap of faith.

The nest was safe, leaving was an unknown quantity, and the path ahead could be fraught with danger.

A voice whispered, *"I will light the way,"* into his mind, and there was the light!

He opened his eyes to find himself perched on the edge of a mighty cliff. If he were to falter....

There was the voice again, *"I will catch thee."*

The eagle took a deep breath and leapt out into the abyss.

He stretched his wings out and soared high above the all, never looking back….

Fly free

No matter where the winds took the eagle, his angel was always there to catch him should he fall.

And fall he did, many a time, always emerging stronger for having survived the experience.

It was then that the eagle realized he'd been conceived out of the very air itself and that he could no more fall than the sun could refuse to shine.

With that he unfurled his wings to their full two meter span and became the mighty eagle he was born to be.

Fly free my friends, fly free.

Days Gone By

Long gone are the days when *all* the snow was as pure as the driven snow, before pollution… before in the name of progress, mankind invented all manner of things that turned the snow grey….

In days of yore, before we sought to cover the planet in concrete, I marveled at the beauty that was snow… how it covered everything in a gentle blanket of white… like dust dropped by the angels… a gift from heaven, one which humanity has sought to spoil, like so many of the other gifts from God.

No more are the days in which our houses did not even have locks, before there were guns and we covered the world in warfare and strife.

As clear as day I see the roads, all of dirt, before everyone had to have a car, before there was so much machinery around us all, destroying life, before cell phones.…

Today I saw myself sitting by the stream near that castle I lived in so long ago, having a picnic with my brother and our families, playing in the water.

I take great comfort in knowing that right now, at this very moment, I am there as well as here.

Part of me prefers that moment to this one.

Along the Banks of the Rio Grande

A young lieutenant fresh from the Point, my brother was always aggressive and pushed his men hard.

This time though, his squadron was caught on the wrong side of the Rio Grande as they raced back to Texas.

The bloodthirsty Indians slaughtered them to a man and stripped them bare, leaving them to rot in the sun.

Two days later we caught up to those very same Indians and destroyed them.

Though, that didn't make bringing his body home any easier.

I miss you little brother, even though we're together both here and there right now.

Be the Lighthouse

Some days the road is lit and the way is easy, other days the path is dark and the going rough. Fear no darkness, be the lighthouse.

The storm will come and there'll be no shelter, stand tall and let your light shine. Be the lighthouse.

It is said that which doesn't destroy you can only make you stronger, free your mind and choose to be the lighthouse.

One thought can change the entire universe.

Peace or war? Love or hate? Who's right and who's wrong? Who owns this or that bit of dirt? Be the lighthouse and everything will sort itself out just fine.

Many will become lost, be the lighthouse and help them find their way.

Wherever you're going, you're getting there. Your path is already before your feet, be the lighthouse, carry the water and bring your light to the places where there are none.

Tune in to your inner vibration and become millions of voices that carry out across all time and space, be that beacon of hope for those who have none. Be the lighthouse and help them find their way home, be the light to guide their way on.

They're out there, right now, looking for you.

As it gets darker, shine brighter, be the lighthouse, become the eternal light… Be the lighthouse.

The storm's coming… there's always a storm coming.

The lighthouse stands tall, pointing the way, always going where it can do the most good.

Who lives, who dies, who makes all of the hard choices? Whose fault is it, who do we blame in the dark of the night? If there's nowhere to hide, where do you run to?

Stop the madness, stop asking questions, stop running, it's time to turn and make a stand. Be the lighthouse.

Nothing is impossible, be the lighthouse.

Pain and suffering abound, become the lighthouse you were born to be and help heal the world. Be the lighthouse.

Many are too lost to even see the light, shine brighter and burn the fog away.

The sun is always there, yet some cannot see. Be the forklift, lift them up into the light and help them to open their eyes. It's all written right there in your destiny, do it. Don't think about it, don't write about it, don't talk about it, don't try and wrap your head around it, just do it. Let go of all of those preconceived notions about yourself and be the lighthouse.

Storms come and go, empires rise and fall, night turns into day, it's all part of the natural order of things. After all, life is a circle, two circles to be precise, infinity, the Infinite, always coming around and going around.

The Infinite talks to everyone, how many listen? Clear your mind and be the lighthouse.

Ideas, great ideas from masters past and present, offer salvation, yet who heeds their words? Why is anyone ever persecuted for thinking or doing something other than the accepted norm? Why fear change?

Be the lighthouse, be the instrument of change, start with yourself and elevate the entire world to be ten times greater than yourself. What a glorious land that would be!

And yet it's all within our grasp right now, all we have to do is choose it.

Wake the others, the time is now.

Miracles happen every day, why not believe in them?

Your world is only limited by the depths of your imagination. Imagine a world filled only with peace, love, and happiness, one where everyone shared all that they had and all that they were, where there are no haves and have nots….

Change your thinking and change the world. Be the lighthouse.

When do we stop blaming, "Them," and start taking responsibility for our own actions? "They," did this to us, "they," did that to us.

Remember when you were a kid and everybody in sight was your best friend? Whatever happened to those days when we all got along? And who's they? Especially when we're all one.

Some children believe in angels and fairy tales, others play make believe and dream of what they'll be when they grow up. Who said you ever had to grow up? I'm going to be a lighthouse when I grow up.

Never let go of your dreams, and never, ever give up.

Why fight over anything when it's all just energy?

What do children know that many adults seem to have forgotten as they seek to acquire and to possess, more?

It's all just a game, have fun with it. Never take anything or yourself too seriously.

Why hoard anything? You can't take it with you. All it does is deprive someone else.

See God in all, uplift them and be the lighthouse.

Let go of the past, let go of what you think your life should be and be the lighthouse.

If everyone were a lighthouse, who would there be to uplift? Let's find out.

What are you waiting for? Get out of your own way and do it!

By killing another, you're killing a part of yourself. Why then do we make war on ourselves?

How many more wars will it take, when will we ever learn?

Be the lighthouse and show them there is a better way to settle our differences.

Clear your mind and clear your karma, be the lighthouse.

How does hurrying about as if the sky were falling help you to evolve? You have to decide for yourself, what's more important, being online and in touch all the time or freeing your mind? Plug into a new reality, the technology of your mind, and put it to work for you.

Yes, it really is that simple, the choice is yours. Everything is as easy as you make it. Be the lighthouse and help others to free themselves before it's too late.

Everyone is special, help them to see it. Some will attack you, not understanding who and what you are. Love them all the same, unconditionally and without hesitation.

You're God, so is everyone and everything else, help them to remember that before they destroy themselves and the world we live on.

Despite whatever wrongs you think they've committed, there's never a good reason to hurt another. Never fault anyone for doing what they feel they have to to survive.

The strength of your own practice will carry you through any adversity.

Be the lighthouse and together we'll change the world.

Sat Nam.

The choices we make

Bound into the symbol for infinity, there is but one real choice.

The pain comes and the mind rails against it, begging for release. Yet if the body is not real, how then is the pain real?

Surrender all attachments as you bow down to the infinite, even to your body, after all it's only a vehicle.

Listen, what's that? The Infinite's talking to you, are you listening?

Dare to Dream

Have you ever walked on the moon?

Have you ever danced in a rainbow?

Have you ever swam in a sea of light, adrift in an ocean of love?

Have you ever seen a place so perfect that it took your breath away and held you rooted in place like a mighty oak? I have, twice….

How then to explain the spirit of Wahe Guru?

It's not a thing you can see or touch, instead it's a way of being, something I carry around with me. I manifest my own happiness from within, I choose to be happy and I am, Wahe Guru!

Things come to me, and I write them down. Does that mean, anything? It all just is, Wahe Guru!

Life is what you make it, enjoy it. Choose to let go, live, love, and walk in the light!

Sat Nam.

Memories to last lifetimes

*M*emories to last lifetimes, friends to always treasure, so many special moments shared with all of them. Where to begin, what to say about this amazing group of people? How could words ever express the myriad of feelings that come to mind as I ponder our experiences high in the desert… the sun coming up over the mesa as we finish our 85th set of yoga….

There exists a bond shared only between those of us that were there, and we didn't all make it. An eagle fell along the way….

Irregardless of what we went in expecting, those three weeks we shared changed our lives forever. I know I for one, have applied a new definition to the word intensive.

Flesh is transitory and so is pain, yet whether it's in your head or real it hurts just the same. Every time one of us was in pain, of any kind, there was always someone right there to lend a helping hand. A shoulder to lean on, someone to talk to in the dark of the night, or anything else you needed.

Voices cry out in the night, and the lighthouse is there, ever ready to answer the call. Be the lighthouse, at any cost to yourself, never refuse another in need.

Sometimes that means something as simple as just playing Frisbee with them, other times it might mean going for a walk with them. Or it might entail helping them to heal the emotional scars of pain they've carried for the last fifty lifetimes, but a lighthouse never backs away from a challenge.

You can do anything you put your mind to, there are no limits, not even the sky.

Until our time there in the desert I had never experienced love, kindness, and compassion on such a scale. Who would have dreamed such things were possible? It had never occurred to me.

The only limits are in your mind, free your mind and free the world.

How profound it all is, what we've become. I for one had no idea what I was in for. Who would have thought? In fact I didn't, I just knew it was the thing to do. Isn't that what it's really all about, following your intuition instead of thinking about it?

Doing, carrying the water, getting up at 3:15am when you REALLY don't want to, that's what it's all about. Shedding attachments, pushing yourself up off the floor one more time, then another, and another, until that buzzer rings, that's what it is to be a lighthouse.

Giving up isn't a part of the path to shuniya, a lighthouse would never give up on themselves or another. There's always hope, even in the darkest hour, in the calm before the storm.

They say it's always darkest right before the storm. Have you looked around lately? It's getting pretty dark, our time is short, and we have much work to do. Be the lighthouse and see it through.

"*God's will be done.*" Not mine, not yours, but God's. No attachments, to outcomes or physical things. It all comes with complete surrender, everything you've ever dreamed of will become yours the moment you no longer want any of it.

Allow the sounds to wash over you as you still your mind and body, let it all go and surrender to the Infinite. "*Ray man eh bidh jog kamaa-o….*" It's all right there, all the answers to every question you've ever had, let go and know the answers.

Tune in to your new reality, all it takes is five little words… "*Ong Namo Guru Dev Namo.*"

Let go and step aside. If you aren't going to trust the Infinite, why'd you even bother to get out of bed?

Wouldn't Becoming Like Eagles be a cool name for a kriya? Or how about Becoming a Lighthouse, because that's really what it's all about.

Scattered though we are, all across the world my dear friends, we're all still together both in my heart and there at the Ghost Ranch. We're timeless and I treasure each and every one of you.

Sat Nam and thank you my blessed friends.

If dolphins ruled the world

I lost a brother at Stalingrad, then again, everybody did. That's what war does, consumes lives with complete neutrality and without compassion.

The war doesn't care who wins or loses or who lives or dies, it all just feeds the cycle of violence so that the war can continue. Who invented war?

At what point did reason no longer prevail and might become right? Having the power to destroy the world is nothing compared to having the power to save the world, or to free your own mind. We as a race have to decide which it will be.

Have you ever wondered, what the world would be like if dolphins ruled the world? There's a reason they don't fiddle with the affairs of men. What do they know that humans don't know? Other than the futility of war, hoarding, and the concept of money along with all of the buying and selling that it entails?

Who invented slavery? It wasn't a dolphin, some human being not only came up with the idea, but then convinced others to go along with it.

Every great society, that has risen however phoenix-like from the ashes of the previous great society, has eventually fallen like a meteor, why?

It all started with a thought.

I mean imagine, somewhere, once upon a time, the first war ever fought was contemplated. Someone not only had the idea, then they went out and did it.

Ever wonder what dolphins are trying to tell us? Maybe, just maybe, it's the most profound words ever uttered on this planet and no human has the ears to hear it. Then again....

How does a dolphin measure wealth? In the abundance of fish? Then again, maybe they're great philosophers trying to figure out how to save humanity and the entire planet from extinction. It's closer to the truth than you realize.

They live very simply, swimming, eating, and mating. Imagine if the average human got that much exercise every day! Why there'd be no time left for work! Wow! What a thought that would be, if we could all spend our day doing what we loved!

"And inhale!"

The first 20 days

"*Ray Man eh Sat Nam, Ray Man eh Sat Nam.*" The sheer profoundness of those words struck me like a thunderbolt, instantly piercing to the utter core of my being. "*Ray Man eh,*" O my mind, "*Sat Nam,*" truth is my identity. "*Ray Man eh, Sat Nam,*" O my mind, truth is my identity! Wahe Guru!

Until I started learning it, I never knew or appreciated the depth of the Ray Man Shabad. I just knew that I liked it. Partly it was cool because Guru Gobind Singh wrote it and he's my guy, but there was something much more to it. I just didn't know what....

Surrendered into what some have called Super Pretzel Pose or Torture Pose, there is no escape. The pain will come, but it's all just in your head. Are you in charge of your mind or is it in charge of you?

The energy flows in an infinite loop, circulating through the body, as you sit bowed before the Infinite.

At first the pain was almost too much to bear, yet I longed for more and kept at it, learning what I needed to stretch out the most before even attempting to get into the posture. Namely everything....

Every day there's less pain, it's easier to get out of the posture, and I always look forward to my, "Bound Time," like it was something a part of me **knew** I needed….

In the beginning the seconds seemed like hours, now the time flies by as I chant along with the Ray Man Shabad. It even takes away a lot of the pain, it's not real anyway, the pain or your head.

If this is what the first 20 days have been like, I wonder where the days to come will take me….

It matters not, it's all a part of my path.

Find yours….

October 9th

October 9th, 2005, in Ottawa, my last full day here.

It's amazing, the twists and turns our path takes in this road called life.

You just hop on a plane and bam, you're somewhere else, catching up with your brothers and sisters, all angels you've met along the way.

The money will come, worry not.

The adventure is in exploring the unknown, take that step outside of your comfort zone, be the lighthouse and shine ever brighter.

Sat Nam.

How much is enough?

*H*ow much is enough? Of anything, how much does one person or one nation need? Certainly not all of it and most definitely not mountains of it, so why is it not shared?

Everyone has something of value, something to contribute to the whole, yet some choose to keep it all for themselves. It's all a house of cards and here comes the wind....

Hold onto your hats, for the world's about to balance itself out. It's been preached for decades and beyond, yet who heeds the warnings? A select few, those who don't fit in or have been branded outcasts by society.

Fear creates that hoarding mentality, fear of lack. Well if you're afraid, you haven't seen nothing yet!

To some it will look like the world is ending, those outcasts though, to them it will be like the first sunrise the world has ever seen. In a way that's what it will be, as the Earth is reborn.

Nature always seeks balance, big animals eating the little animals, survival of the fittest and all that. Humans, as a race, haven't quite mastered that concept yet. Those outcasts, they've got it down, they're called lighthouses.

They say nothing lasts forever. Of course it does. You can never truly destroy anything no matter how hard you try. It's all energy, it just changes form. No matter how much force is applied, irregardless of what manner of destruction is applied to it, no force man can apply to a thing will ever totally destroy it. It will always exist somewhere, as something.

Violence has its place, everything does, but what about the wisdom to use it properly? We lost it during the rush for progress, covering the planet with concrete as humanity multiplied exponentially.

You have to smash a walnut to open it just as you split firewood before you put it in the fireplace. There are of course exceptions to every rule, but the principal is the same. Nature is going to rebalance itself and it's going to be the most violent thing this Earth has seen since its creation.

Or not, it's all up to you, right now. Choose to be the lighthouse and save the world, or not. You have free will, use it.

It's not about your neighbor, it's all about you. You, right now, can save the entire world with but a thought. Be the lighthouse.

How then, to be the lighthouse, you ask? Everything starts with a thought, even the universe did.

Shedding attachments which no longer serve you is a place to begin. Persons, places, things, desires, perceived needs, it's all just an illusion, you don't really need any of it, and you can never truly lose anything, so why worry about it?

Money, power, anything that can be craved can and will pull you from your path if you but let it. That's how the game works, but you knew that going in, the real question is, who knows it now? Ah, there's those outcasts again, working to help the very people they didn't fit in with. Then again, that's what a lighthouse does….

Wahe Guru!

Sponsorship

Everything has a sponsor these days, a name on a thing, to promote, to advertise, in the pursuit of profit.

Here's a few basics some might have forgotten along the way—

Life, brought to you by God.

Kundalini Yoga, brought to you by Yogi Bhajan.

Enlightenment, brought to you by yourself and God. Remember your partnership?

Everyone plays the game, some more seriously than others. Some play to win, unwittingly competing against themselves, others spread the light. I guess it's all just about which game you're playing….

The pain will come for you, I promise. Are you going to stand up to it, or crumble before it? The choice is yours.

When did it become fashionable to be so critical? It not only reinforces the not good enough mentality, but the separatist theory as well. It's not a contest, we're all in this together.

Does your left arm try and defeat the right? No, they work together, now if we could all just do that, think what we could accomplish!

Wahe Guru!

Chant now

C hant now, out into the Infinite, and for all time. Chant so the angels can hear, remember, God's listening, are you?

Vibrate down to the depths of your soul as the Golden Lady chants, *"Ong Namo Guru Dev Namo."*

Water falls from the sky, yet many go thirsty, why?

Carry the water so that no one ever goes thirsty again.

Be the lighthouse.

Vibrate and the entire universe vibrates with you.

All can be golden, yet how many are willing to do the work it takes to get there? Show them the way, be the lighthouse.

Sat Nam.

Eagles and trains

On a train bound for Toronto, our eagle left his angel behind. No regrets, over any of his choices, decisions, or anything else.

The entirety of his existence had led him to that single point where he sat watching a light drizzle fall.

Not knowing what was to come, he eagerly awaited whatever the future might bring him.

Blessings, nothing but blessings….

He'd been to the mountain, met the Golden Lady, and even had his own personal angel. He'd been to heaven and no longer feared death, or anything else for that matter.

Thank you God, bless you!

Wahe Guru!

Chasing ghosts

Build it high to stand for all time, to show the next ten thousand generations the futility of war.

Wars come and wars go as do the young people who are consumed in them.

Soldiers are awarded medals, what about the families of those who don't come home?

Madness, sheer madness.

Paranoia is destroying our world. Suspicion and fear? Of what, ourselves? What's next, your right foot attacking the left?

Wake up and stop killing your brothers and sisters.

Be the lighthouse, be the beacon of hope and light the way to peace in our world. It can happen, all with a thought.

Be the lighthouse now and for all time.

The ghosts of our war dead wander the world, seeking absolution for the deeds they've committed against their brothers and sisters.

Be the lighthouse and help the world to remember history and to finally learn the futility of war.

Be the lighthouse and help guide the ghosts on their way home.

Sat Nam.

Angels and Eagles

I nextricably intertwined, the lives of these creatures of flight. One soars, the other moves by sheer force of will, just a thought and it is so….

I'm blessed to know my angel personally, open your eyes and find yours.

After all these years, across countless lifetimes, I finally comprehend love.

It transcends all, love, the true nature of the universe. A state of mind, THE way to be, it encompasses all and excludes none.

Freedom with responsibility, blessing and accepting all without question, caring for another above the needs of the self, now that is love.

Things come and go in our lives, people, places, careers, helping us along on our way, but angels are forever. At least, my bond with mine is….

Eternal beings of light are they, ever present and ever conscious, lifting us up, being the lighthouse.

Bless you God, my partner in creation, for this miracle called life.

Wahe Guru!

Ray Man eh

"*Ray Man eh, Sat Nam.*" Oh my mind, truth is my identity.

I carry a piece of an angel with me, she gave it to me freely, asking nothing for herself.

In return I gave her a piece of my heart. She carries it in her heart as she helps to heal the world.

Talk about being the lighthouse! She is my lighthouse, always there for me, shining her light.

We can never truly be apart, no matter the distance, yet I miss her nevertheless.

"Sat Nam," truth is my identity.

I can see her with my waking eyes, I feel the warmth of her touch, how could I possibly miss what is right here with me?

Come what may, we will always be together, shoulder to shoulder against the storm.

Sat Nam.

Who's awake?

Who's awake and who's asleep?

Homeless lay on the street corner, being stepped over by the society who forgot them.

Who's asleep and who's awake?

Most are asleep, be the lighthouse, shine bright and rouse them from their unconscious life. Help them to rediscover their true angelic nature, help them to see God in all, help them so they can help themselves and in turn spread the light.

We....

We, is the meaning of life. If we would all remember that we are all one, we would solve all our problems.

Be the lighthouse and see it done, change the world by your very presence.

Carry the water and be the lighthouse.

Sat Nam.

All along the shore

Waves crash as the sea roils with all its might, as if to say, "I AM GOD!!!" No one but the willow tree listens.

It waves its branches, replying, "I too am God."

The sea pounds on, heralding the approaching storm....

We....

The shore gives way as nature seeks balance, cleansing itself of the ills inflicted upon it.

The unwary venture too near, the willow tree stands calm, scant yards from the shore. It understands that "we" is the meaning of life and it fears nothing.

The willow tree sings as it shelters me against the cold, "*The greatest secret ever told, timeless, ageless are we, for we are all God. Tell your brothers, tell your sisters.*"

The waves grow taller, more violent, emphasizing the trees point.

It's time to move on, it's getting darker and there's work to be done....

The masses huddle under the tree, too busy to hear its song. Be the lighthouse and help them all to hear.

Be the lighthouse.

Faith manages

There's always hope, never let anyone tell you otherwise.

Even in your most desperate hour, God watches over you.

Someone once said, "Faith manages." How much faith do you have?

Enough to travel to the middle of the desert to become a yoga teacher?

Enough to leave behind all that you have and all that you know?

Enough to give up the life you knew, all because God said, "Let go, trust me."

Faith manages.

Just because you can't see your destination, that doesn't mean it's not there. I can't see California right now, but I know it's there. I can't see the storm, but that doesn't mean it's not coming. God told me it was….

Faith manages.

Against the Odds came first, a struggle against the impossibly impossible. They survived, to face the storm, The Approaching Storm….

Who survives depends on the few who are willing to do the work, those who willingly sacrifice all that they have and just carry the water.

So much of what I write revolves around storms. Why?

"You know why," echoes through my mind as tears form at the edges of my eyes. "NO!"

"No what?" "The world doesn't have to be destroyed."

"No it doesn't. But if you don't take care of it, you will destroy it, not me."

Sigh

No pressure there….

"No, not really, remember, you're just the guy with the bucket of water? Be the lighthouse and all that?" *Smiles*

"No attachments, no worries." *Smiles* "I remember. Is anybody ever going to read any of this?"

"What do you think?" "I'd like to think so, but isn't that just wishful thinking?"

"Sounds to me like that's faith managing." *Laughs*

Rereading a few pages of what I referred to as TAS, I ran across these four words—fear is a choice….

Things come to me and I write them down, my partnership with God. It's as simple as that.

Fear is a choice. I've chosen faith, in myself and in God. I don't consciously write for myself. Yes, it's very meditative and therapeutic for me and I am conscious of what I write. When I'm relaxed and open, it just comes to me, though, I don't try and force it or direct it where I think it should go.

"*That's how it's supposed to work.*" "Cool." "*Very.*"

"Okay, so then what?" "*Meditate, do yoga, write, and I'll take care of everything else.*"

"Sat Nam! Wahe Guru!"

"Thank you God, for being my friend and partner in all that I do. Thank you for helping me to see God in myself and in everything else. Thank you for everything. Bless you."

"*Sat Nam.*"

Forgiveness can heal anything, faith can move mountains, love can change the entire universe, and you can be as happy as you want, all with a thought. So what will it be?

My question for you is, who was I just talking to? Myself? God?

Both.

The willow tree

*R*ound and round go the unwise, ever repeating the same cycles of life as they scurry to and fro, hustling and bustling about in the concrete jungle.

A light rain falls, attempting to cool their rush. They hurry on, struggling to make time.

How pray tell do you make time?

Run too fast and you'll miss the rain singing, "*Ong Namo Guru Dev Namo.*"

Can you hear it? The willow tree does….

Free your mind and free the world.

In pursuit of the light

*T*he journey doesn't end here, this is only just the beginning.

Many are already scared, wait till all the lights go out and the world goes berserk.

We'll meet again, in a place where no shadows fall, I promise you my friends.

The dawn approacheth, in the meantime, be the lighthouse.

They say it's always darkest right before the dawn, well, it's about to get really dark….

But then again, how can it really get much darker? It's all about perception, especially now as we transition into the Aquarian Age.

The pursuit of profit seems all the more pointless now….

Soon it will all be about the pursuit of the light….

Akal

*B*ound to race about, born to space, the undying choose a mortal existence for their own evolution.

Bound to the Infinite, each other, everything, we sacrifice our limitless nature to be limited.

God is everything, everywhere, as am I.

Why am I cutting down all of my trees, why am I polluting my own drinking water? Why am I robbing myself? Why do I have guns? To protect me from myself?

Instead of fighting, let's all do some yoga together.

Come on, come here and sit down with me and let's tune in.

We're all one, you all know each other. The world is our living room, so stop messing it up!

Storms

I don't "try" to write, it comes to me, seemingly of its own accord.

Shuniya! Ah—ha! It's when I relax, shuniya if you will, that it comes through me. Wahe Guru! Life is really a quest for shuniya....

A hard rain falls, lightning flashes across the sky and the trees blow as yet another storm coalesces. No surprise there....

Thunder echoes across the land, the storm shouting, "Here I come!"

It's coming for me, and you too.

Soon the land will be cleansed and the flowers will rise anew...but not just yet.

Lightning strikes into the ground, the storm accentuating its point, "Here I am!" We all see it....

The storm understands though. It has surrendered, letting itself be blown about by the wind. No particular place to go, just going.

It's dark now, the storm long since fallen quiet, come and gone like the wind....

They'll keep coming though, until we hear and heed their message....

The power of thought

*E*verybody loves cliffhangers, a big buildup of suspense and drama and then they leave you hanging. But then we tune back in to see how the story unfolds, we keep turning those pages.

You are the storm.

Every storm dissipates, achieves shuniya if you will. If we all reach shuniya, there'll be no more storms.

"Our thoughts, words, and actions create the weather?"

"In part yes. It's possible to make rain, yes?" "Yes."

"A few hundred people chanting and meditating can produce a nice gentle rain, yes?"

"Yes."

"Imagine the creative power of the thoughts of a million angry people…five million…a hundred…."

"There'll be no shelter here."

"Be the lighthouse and there will. You always have a choice, you yourself can help determine how difficult the transition is."

The greatest lie ever told

*T*here's a great many illusions in this game called life, none more so than the separatist theory.

The perceived need for money plays right into that belief.

You need money to buy things. Why? Separatism.

You, me, us, them, they, all different ways of defining the same thing—the mistaken belief that we are all separate individuals.

A strong enough crisis of faith will cause you to almost lose your mind. No worries, no attachments, nothing but complete and total surrender can save you.

The more you grow, the greater the challenges you shall face....

"Tell me about it!"

"Okay, I will. You yourself declared, to me, that you wanted to grow, the easy part's over. Now comes the real work."

"Great."

"Yes it is, do you realize how far you've come?"

"Far enough to about lose my mind today."

"Oh just wait! You're only writing about it now, wait till you teach it!"

"Sat Nam."

"Just wait till you see what's in store for you. You know, you just don't want to admit it. What are you afraid of?"

"Wanting a thing won't bring me the thing."

"Detachment yes, but you can't deny who and what you are."

"I'm just a guy, the guy with the bucket of water."

"You're more than just that."

"Who almost lost his mind today."

"That you did, and you want to know why?"

"Lamenting the past, choices I made and the money my decisions cost me."

"But look at how you've grown from those experiences."

"True, but at the time it was the money I didn't have and the bills that I did that really weighed me down. I couldn't see past it."

"And now?"

Sigh "I'm having a conversation with God/myself."

"That doesn't answer the question."

"Well sure it does, that means I'm open and relaxed enough to hear."

"Sat Nam."

"Sat Nam."

"Remember, darkness balances the light. Night turns into day and so on."

"Yeah, and it was that balance that I lost track of. Two of the costlier investments, I had to make, because that was what finally helped me to let go of that burning desire for money that had possessed me for so many years."

"Aren't you being a bit harsh on yourself?"

"Correction, that was where I learned the true cost of working so much overtime, what it did to me and how little I really gained."

"The money will come my friend, keep on writing, share it and what you know with the world. Be the lighthouse."

"Sat Nam, bless you God, and thank you."

Demons

*T*he further up the mountain you go, the tougher the demons get.

Sigh

Floating along, illusions tear at the mind, doing their best to pull me from the path. At times I can't even see the path, other times it's as clear as day.

Right now, the sun shines down, warming my face in the cool mountain air.

It's clear, I can see for miles, I just can't see the demons. They lurk here and there, hiding in the shadows, waiting to ambush me....

I've noticed, that after I do Bound, they can't touch me. Beforehand, it's open season on me... all the more incentive to surrender first thing in the morning.

Demons don't do sadhana, but they're up, waiting for you. They never sleep....

At least in the dark, I can't see the illusions either....

It's profoundly calming, this Bound Lotus. Today was my 35th day, and there'll be no demons.

Not that there's demons in the classic sense of the word, distractions, unchecked emotions that take root and hold sway over me. Bound brings the deepest calm imaginable, oneness, shuniya, and it strengthens my connection to the Infinite. It also restores my faith, a thousandfold....

I can feel it, healing my entire body at a cellular level, broadening my awareness as it elevates my consciousness.

The day will come, when there'll be no more demons, but until then I have my angel, my dear friends, Bound and a host of other tools to help get me where I'm going.

Someone once said, "If it was easy, everyone would do it." Well it is easy, it's just all in how you look at it. Perception determines your reality.

Do you set out to do something or to try to do something? Which will get your further, trying or doing?

The energy courses through me, hands to feet, feet to hands, as I fold myself up and bow down before the Infinite. Doing, not trying.

Yes failure is still a part of doing, it's a part of the learning process, but if you try once, fail, and then give up, what have you accomplished? You've let the demons win....

I'll be in the snow soon, I can see it. It's getting colder and I've still got a long ways to go....

The mountain and I have a most unique relationship. I've made it my own and it tolerates my presence. All I leave are footsteps....

It seems not to mind, at times I even hear it singing. Or maybe that's just the wind....

On the other hand though, it doesn't care about the demons either. They're my demons, they don't bother the mountain, but they sure do their best to bother me.

Bound, banishes the demons, for almost an entire day... I've just now realized it....

There's pain, and a lot of it at that. I won't sugar coat it, at first it almost drove me mad, but every day it gets easier and I'm far more flexible than ever before.

So here I am, barefoot in the cold. At least I have a jacket on, and my head's covered too....

No demons today, it's onward and upward, though, I can't see where the path goes....

The wind howls, as if to say, "*This way....*"

Another day, another day closer to my destination.

Keep on climbing and reach yours.

Sat Nam.

The mountain

*C*omputers are curious things, rather like humans they are....

There're no storms on the mountain, or computers for that matter, she doesn't tolerate either. It snows though, a lot too, I can see it....

Some days I wonder what's at the top of the mountain, other days it takes all I can muster just to keep going, to push myself up one more time, to take one more step, then another.

The air's thin up here, at times my lungs burn as they strain for breath. Either way, I'll keep going....

When the demons come for me, it gets awfully lonely on the mountain. That's usually when I fall, hard and far too....

Then there's days like today, not only am I calm and centered but I'm surrounded by friends as well. Not in the physical sense of the word, but I can see and hear them. Angels and eagles, encouraging me, offering support and guidance as I journey on....

Talk about the road less traveled! This is like the road never traveled. I guess that makes sense, it's my path, not anyone else's....

Not even a footprint, no trace whatsoever, of anyone else ever having been up here before me.

The mountain is timeless, a true master of time and space.

Now, I "know" the way, when the demons come, I get lost and wander aimlessly. All the more reason to surrender.

There's no food up here, yet I don't go hungry, or lack anything for that matter.

When the demons come, that's when I worry, about all kinds of things but namely money.

Money has no use up here, and there're no cars or technology of any kind.

The demons though, they bring the illusions with them. It's my mountain though, just like they're my demons....

The mountain II

*I*t's a clear day, there'll be no demons today, not for me that is. They're out there though, waiting....

Everyone has their own demons, their own hills to climb....

It's even colder today, but now I have a thick coat and boots on, gifts from my friend....

The higher I go, the colder its gets, the bigger the demons are....

Today I can even see the top, just not the way, no matter, I know the way.

The killing fields are far behind me now. In fact, if all goes well, I'll be in the snow soon.

BAM!!!!!

Silly me, the road to shuniya requires constant effort, there are no magic pills, no wave of the hand and instantly you're there. Well, maybe someday, but not today, not for me.

They came for me, full force, knocking me down and sending me flying back down the hill. Jealousy....

I tumble and slide, the lights go out, all because of a half a minutes worth of thoughts. Jealousy leads to anger, that's when I fell.

Eventually I slid to a stop, having lost a lot of ground. But, it's warmer now, the sun's out, and, I can see the way. That's the good thing about falling....

I chant a lot these days. I love it, and the demons hate it. I'm particularly fond of the Ray Man Shabad. It's energizing and incredibly healing, among other things.

So back up we go....

Friends

*T*here're no guarantees in this thing called life and Bound alone won't keep the demons away forever. Not demons this size....

A brief conversation with the dearest of friends can inspire you to amazing heights.

If you're not centered, it's just as easy to get thrown right off the mountain entirely.

The mountain of course is a metaphor for my path and the demons are just those stumbling blocks that pop up along the way. And I do feel that Bound is the ultimate pop up blocker, but you can't rely on one tool alone. You have hundreds, use them.

What was once the dearest of friends came and went without a trace, never to be heard from again. She left behind the most precious of gifts, my writing.

Many things inspire me, but that was where it all began, creating for an audience of one.

It's grown since then and I've made new friends, even an angel befriended me....

Some days I fall down, a lot, but I always get up and keep on going, thanks largely to the strength and support of my friends.

Dark days come, and I fall hard and fast, but I never give up, not on myself or hope.

Keep pushing yourself up off the ground and be the lighthouse, the world needs you.

Sat Nam

It can happen

*F*oreboding talk, of lighthouses, storms, demons, and mountains, where does it all lead? Ideally, to shuniya.

I hope, to be able to help people, to heal the world....

If there truly is no such thing as limits, then it can happen. If I can think of it, it can happen.

If I tell just one person, and they tell two people, who in turn tell four people, who tell eight people, and so on, we'll create a wave of light and elevate the entire planet. Carry the water and see it done.

It's contagious, you catch it from someone, this drive to be the lighthouse. In this world of quick fixes there are no shortcuts, you can't take it like a pill, you have to do the work.

Fall in love with the process of freeing your mind and you'll be the lighthouse. Stop running around, sit down and take control of your mind. It's yours, who's in charge, you or it? You decide....

You have all the tools, use them.

I'm just a guy, but I know I can make a difference and you can too. It all has to start somewhere, be that catalyst for change, be the lighthouse and change the world.

The sun will shine, who will see it? It's not for me to decide, but if I can bring a smile to just one person's face, change their day, or even help them to think in a new way, you can too. We're all in this together, this thing called life, relax, tune in and be the lighthouse.

Hope, faith, dreams, everyone has them to varying degrees.

The pain comes, the arms hurt, yet, somewhere, somehow, you find the strength to push yourself up off the floor one more time. Then another, and another. How?

By not giving up, by knowing you can do it. Just once more, come on, push, push!

Whatever happened to that can do, pioneer spirit? Did it become buried under mountains of technology? Or did we sell it to the highest bidder?

It's still there, somewhat forgotten but not gone, not yet. Rekindle the flames, help the world to push itself up off the floor, one more time, then another, and another.

Surrender yes, but never give up. Carry the water and see it done, in our lifetime, for all time. Be the lighthouse.

Sat Nam.

It just comes to me

*I*t just comes to me, and I write it down. I don't really try and figure it all out, wrap my head around it if you will. I did at first, I think, but then it didn't come to me, my head was too cluttered up with my own thoughts and such.

If I can do it, you can do it too.

It's a product of doing yoga and meditation, Kundalini Yoga to be specific. That's where it really started to flow, as it became easier to relax into the flow. It just is.

I don't really think about it, I just enjoy the process. It's deeply therapeutic and incredibly healing for me. Some of it makes me sad, it's also very inspiring though as it encourages me to relax.

It's very meditative, yet I have to be relaxed for it to come through. Quite the interesting relationship the two have, especially given how profoundly relaxing the writing is.

It's a deeper relaxation as it comes through. There's still ups and downs, things that knock me off my center, but I'm far calmer and stiller than I've ever been before. And I have the tools to bring myself back to center now. We grow up without them....

I don't think about why I write, I just do. I'm just the messenger, the guy with the bucket of water if you will.

There's more than enough for everyone, let's all share it. That's what being the lighthouse is all about, thinking of others not yourself. After all, they are you.

Peace be with us all, bless you.

Sat Nam.

Love

*I*f you love someone, tell them.

When you hold someone, hold them for all time.

Doom and gloom aside, the sun will shine through it all.

Sat Nam, truth is my identity.

My highest truth is that I am God and so are you.

Wahe Guru, I am in ecstasy when I experience the Indescribable Wisdom.

Be the lighthouse and help the world to experience Wahe Guru for themselves.

Sat Nam.

Against the odds

Odds? What odds? Who said it couldn't be done? Push yourself up off the floor one more time just to prove them wrong, then do it once for yourself, once for God, then once for....

Even when your arms are shaking to the point of collapsing, you can do it one more time, I know you can.

Believe in yourself and the world will too.

There's no such thing as insurmountable odds, it just makes for a greater challenge and provides a much greater sense of accomplishment when you see it done.

Infinity's a lot, but anything is possible.

Everything is energy, yet here we are having this existence.

Storms come and go as do people. Times change, as does the world. We have seven years to go and oh what a show it's going to be! Wahe Guru!

It's said that knowing is half the battle.

I know that we as a race can do this, now, in our lifetime, if we all just work together.

Even just a few lighthouses here and there, that's how it all starts. It'll hurt and even be too much for some to bear, but I know you can do it.

Life just is, life, make it what you choose. Be the lighthouse so everyone can choose.

See it done and we all win.

Peace and love....

Day 40

What a thing this Bound Lotus is.

Forty down, only 960 to go. Then again, I may never stop.

Today, I stood on the brink and looked into the abyss. I saw myself loosing control….

Things don't always go our way and ever bigger challenges arise. Not just money, but keeping our cool when the entire world crashes down around us.

Forty days… a lifetime to go.

Ideas take form, thanks largely to the serenity that Bound brings. It all takes shape, so many things come together at last.

Now if I could just fall asleep! Ideas run through my head, anticipation, knowing it will all work out.

Yet here I lay, pen in hand instead of sleeping.

I yawn, more ideas yet to note.

What a day this day 40 has been. Thankfully, I have the tools, lest I lose my mind….

War

War wouldn't exist if everyone refused to fight.

How many more kids have to end up face down in the sand, and how many more times do I have to ask that?

"*You* don't have to do anything."

"You know what I mean."

"*Yes I do, dwelling on it isn't going to help you do anything about the situation now is it?*"

"Of course not." *smiles*

"*Good. Now, shuniya.*"

"Yes?"

"*Shuniya, now.*"

"Right, yes, I thought we were going to talk about shuniya?"

"*It's a course of action, not a topic for discussion.*"

"Meaning I need a little detachment, thank you."

"*Don't think so much, relax into shuniya so we can create.*"

"I know, I was worrying about money again today, thinking about what I had left."

"*Dwelling on the negative won't help you now will it?*"

"Nope, nor will it help me improve my cash flow!"

Laughter

"Bless you God, thank you, Sat Nam."

"*Peace my friend, relax into shuniya and let it come, it will. Dwell in darkness no more.*"

Demand

*I*t's all a learning experience.

Instead of more fuel efficient cars or adding extra lanes to reduce traffic, how about fewer cars?

Everything is a learning experience.

The price of oil goes up, the price of oil goes down.

The price of gas goes up, and eventually it goes back down again.

Right now, supply is down and demand is up.

What's the demand like for lighthouses?

I'm going to go do some Bound Lotus, maybe I'll find out....

When the time comes

*I*nterestingly enough, what I found instead was shuniya.

Day 46 of Bound Lotus.

The universe talks to me, and I'm still enough to hear it.

At last, this day, I've quit chasing about searching for ways to make money. It'll come....

Worrying about it only makes matters worse, and it definitely won't help me relax into shuniya.

My writing is a gift and I know I need to explore that more, to develop it and to help people. That's my goal.

The demand for lighthouses is up, way up.

There's no price tag on a lighthouse. You can't buy one, but one will be there for you when the time comes.

Halfway

It is said that knowing is half the battle. Well, I know I'm a lighthouse, so does that mean that I'm halfway to wherever it is that I'm going? By the way, where am I going?

I'm on the road to shuniya!

Sat Nam!

I saw myself today, returning to the place of my birth, or rebirth as it were. A fertile valley, high in the mountains where I first experienced Wahe Guru....

The dawn approaches, take my hand and climb the mountain with me.

Bask in the light, let it warm your soul.

Fear no darkness, you are the lighthouse.

Bless you.

Sat Nam

Deer

A herd of deer nibble on the grass, unfettered by human "progress."

The deer understand, there's eight of them, roaming free, taking care of each other.

More than likely, it's an entire family, several generations worth, living and traveling together.

They wander about the fields that cover an ancient civilization, caring, not about the current "civilization" but about each other.

Sure, they keep their distance, and for good reason too—they know something that we don't.

Deer walk or run everywhere they go. They live outdoors, living off of the land itself. Such beautiful creatures….

We could learn a lot from deer. How to run like the wind & survive…

Build it high

G ather 'round the campfire brothers and sisters, Lanette, build it high for all to see.

It's getting dark and the world needs our help.

That's what a lighthouse does, always going where it's the darkest, where they can do the most good.

Don't stop until the entire universe can see the light.

No more dire warnings or ominous talk, just a reminder—carry the water, be the messenger of peace and hope—be the lighthouse.

And I'll keep on saying it…

Be the lighthouse…

Be the lighthouse…

Be the lighthouse.

Do it for your brothers, for your sisters, for the children and the next ten thousand generations. Fear no darkness, be the lighthouse.

Bless you.

Sat Nam.

The wind told me so

Whispers on the wind.

Do you hear it? Few do….

Of my things, my notebook and pen are among my most cherished. They are but things.

Still, if all I have are just those two things, I know I'm a rich man.

It may yet come to that, and you know what, I'm pretty okay with that.

Then again….

Whispers on the wind….

It'll all work out, the wind told me so.

I walked away from a lot, everything, nothing, a cubicle.

"It's in the sacrifice that we grow."

That was over three months ago. If I didn't know better I'd be worried that the money was about to run out, but I'm not and it won't. The wind told me so.

Have faith and hear the wind, it talks to you too....

Blessings

*L*aying in the grass next to a lazy river, my cares float away....

Abundance is on it way downstream, I have but to reach out and grab it.

Wahe Guru!

All my needs are met before I even know I have them. How's that for a blessing?

Wahe Guru!

Freedom brings time for reflection and relaxation, switching gears to being a lighthouse.

When it comes, it will happen all in a rush, are you ready?

Ever greater challenges await, what will you create?

Light and lots of it, is what the world needs, not more distractions.

If it is all just a game, then how do you win?

Then again, not all games have "winners" and "losers." This could be one such game, where there are no clearly defined rules, or even one where we make up the rules as we go along.

It all just is....

Surrender pose

*I*n the beginning, I understood why some had nicknamed it torture pose, this Bound Lotus, but now I think of it as surrender pose, because that's what it is for me, surrender.

Today is Day 55 for me. Not only can I feel it healing my entire body on a cellular level, but it's healing my soul as well.

Folded up as I chant along with a most magical version of the Ray Man Shabad, there's no where to run, no where to hide. It's all right in the open....

There's no escape, only surrender.

Nothing is ever to be undertaken lightly, least of all this Bound Lotus.

The warm-ups alone are more exercise than many kriyas and by comparison, getting into the position is the easy part! It's holding it that can be the most challenging, particularly in the beginning.

At first it hurt so bad my mind screamed, begging for release. It HURT!!!!

I didn't stop though and the pain faded, I can't even remember when, I just know that I'll keep on doing it. I remember how excited I was the first time I wrapped my fingers all the way around both toes! Wahe Guru!

It's been 55 days and already I'm a completely different person. Everything has changed, I'm calmer now than what I've ever been in my entire life!

Everybody can do some version of it, using modifications and or props. I'm blessed with a fair bit of flexibility, it's increased a thousandfold since I started doing Kundalini Yoga. It's just in the doing, moving from a human being to a human doing.

I'm just a guy with a bucket of water. The water is the message.

Be the lighthouse.

I can't wait to see what Day 56 brings!

Wahe Guru!

I am a teacher

See yourself laying by a slow moving river, let all your cares just float away.

Feel your body sinking down into the Earth, let it all go.

It's a beautiful day out, hear the leaves falling from the trees.

Relax and let go of your body.

Hear the wind whispering to you….

I now know what I was put on this Earth to do—to help people.

In that moment, I realized that I didn't care if I never made another dollar in my entire life. God will take care of me, the wind told me so.

Sat Nam.

Be the lighthouse.

War games

I got mad at a thing as innocuous as a game, then again, life is a game,

War isn't a game played only with toy soldiers, this night last, the war was in my mind.

I got so angry, so irate, that I gave up on myself and quit. Rather than keeping on, I took the easy way out. No excuses, I admit what I did.

You can't quit life though, it doesn't solve anything. There's no magic reset button for life, but what if there was?

If there is a next time, I'll approach the thing that angered me differently, if at all.

By that same token you can't measure your success against that of another. Apples and oranges.

Least likely of all is knowing what each other came here to accomplish.

None of that changes the fact that I quit even trying to try. I quit altogether.

The challenges are getting bigger. Pass one, the next one is even bigger. In this case it's a snowball effect, growing and growing.

It's in the pushing ourselves back up off the floor that we truly grow, namely never giving up.

Decidedly over the edge, especially for me. Looking back on it now, I'm unable to decide if I was more upset at the thing that upset me or disappointed in my reaction to it. No, the latter....

As the challenges get greater, keep rising to the occasion, shine through and be the lighthouse.

Come on, let's do some yoga together.

Triumph

The pain cannot be real as I know I am not my body, Bound Lotus has proven that beyond a shadow of a doubt.

The strength of your own personal sadhana (ie spiritual practice) will carry you through any adversity.

When your arms are shaking to the point of collapse and you're about to fall on your head, but you dig deep and push yourself up off the floor one more time, that's when the triumph comes and you transcend the pain and the physical.

Belief in the pain gives it life.

Believe in the light, make it your own and be the lighthouse.

Sat Nam.

Inspiration

H ave you held in your eyes a place so beautiful, a moment so perfect that you never wanted to leave? A land of golden sunsets, where the weather is always perfect....

It exists, in my mind, I can see it right now. I carry it with me wherever I go.

It's been quite some time since my notebook, pen and I last got together. Old friends that are always there for me, just waiting for me to pick them up.

In the dark of the night, what inspires you to be the lighthouse?

For me it's the darkness itself, that, and an overwhelming desire to help people, to be the lighthouse. I'm just the messenger, the guy with the bucket of water.

The sun always rises, never, ever forget that.

Inspiration… it all starts with but a thought, one that propels some to greatness.

Be the lighthouse and inspire the entire world to create peace in our time. It all begins with a thought....

Be the lighthouse, carry the water and bring light to the entire world.

Be the lighthouse.

Creating

We have a date to create, the four of us do, me, God, my pen and my notebook.

When I'm too distracted, too, "busy," we don't create. What's more important than doing God's work?

Being the lighthouse is God's work. I couldn't ask for a better boss!

It will come, in time, money among other things.

I left my job almost four months ago, knowing that the universe would provide for me. It's coming, I know it is....

All I have to do is carry the water, be the messenger, and God will take care of everything else. All in all a pretty good deal if you ask me!

Wahe Guru!

Peace be with you my friends and bless you God!

Sat Nam

Creating II

*I*llness gives pause, as to the cause... *what my thoughts have created... dwelling on the irrelevant as they'd been....*

Our thoughts create, this weekend past, mine created dis-ease, illness in my physical form. It passes as I reorient myself to the task at hand, that of being a lighthouse and being about my father's business.

I read, today, an old email from a dear friend, about inspiration.

She's the reason this book exists. It was her urging and encouragement that gave me the drive to share this with the world. I remember how she said it was a gift from God and was meant to be shared....

Bless you my friend and fellow lighthouse!

Sat Nam

The light is coming

*D*ay 65 of Bound Lotus....

Winter approaches, the wind howls and the leaves fall from the trees. Just like with the Earth, the season is changing.

The interesting thing is, I no longer see the darkness, all I see is the light.

Even in the dark, the light is still there and *that* is what I see, not the darkness.

In a way, it all relates to the question of whether the glass is half full or half empty.

The light is always there, you just have to be able to see it.

And that is what we're all about, helping to bring forth that awakening.

No, no more ominous talk or foreboding warnings of dire circumstances, the light is coming.

The light is coming…

The light is coming…

The light is coming…

Sat Nam

Be the lighthouse.

Five words

"*Ong Namo Guru Dev Namo*," Five words that will change not only the entire world but the course of our existence if we but let them.

It translates as, "I bow to the subtle divine wisdom, the divine teacher within."

If we all chanted it together and tuned into that divine wisdom right now, we would end all suffering and strife on our planet. We could at long last all live in peace and harmony together.

Sit down here with me my brothers and sisters, gather 'round the campfire. Lanette, build it high, the entire world is coming over this evening.

Sit down with us my friends and let's do some yoga together.

"Ong Namo Guru Dev Namo."

Five little words that have the power to change everything. Bow to the divine wisdom and nothing will ever be the same again.

In fact, you'll be a lighthouse....

Corners

We've turned a corner, you and I have my friend, together we're going to change the world, one person at a time.

The very fact that you're reading this means that change has already begun.

That's where it all starts, how the light spreads, from one person to another.

That's what a lighthouse does, carries the water, i.e. the message, to everyone the world over.

Yes, that's a tall order, but nothing's impossible and not even the sky's the limit.

Healing the world is as easy as we make it. If we choose right now, in this very instance, we can end all violence, suffering and hunger on this planet, our home.

Our brothers and sisters are sleeping on street corners, bathing in ditches and scrounging food from the garbage, not to mention killing each other.

We have in our hands the power to end it all right now, before it's too late, before we destroy ourselves, and usher in the greatest time of peace and prosperity our world has ever known.

Which will it be? Only time will tell, I've chosen the light, to be the lighthouse and to help any way I can....

Seeing

I can't see the top of the mountain but I know I'm getting there, even if it doesn't always feel like I'm getting anywhere.

I get distracted or upset and get pulled off my center, off the path as it were, away from shuniya.

No matter what though I always keep pushing myself up off the floor. Kundalini Yoga is my salvation, it's become my life, who and what I am....

I just can't keep retreating into technoland, into my computer. Yes it's a useful tool, but I can't live inside of it.

Life exists out here in the real world, not as a series of ones and zeroes inside of a machine. It is all energy though, be it the electricity that runs our computers or the energies that run our bodies, the most perfect machine ever devised....

It doesn't always feel like it, but I know I'm getting there and so are you.

Come on, sit down here with me by the fire and let's do some yoga together.

"Ong Namo Guru Dev Namo."

Soar

*S*eeing an eagle is always a good sign, a good omen if you believe in such things.

This one called out to me, announcing its presence as it circled high above the valley, floating on the invisible hands of God.

It drifts about, riding high, as if it can see the wind itself!

Gunshots echo from the ridges, deer hunters about their business.

The eagle understands, having mastered flight and so much more.

Its screech is unmistakable, a reminder to let go and soar.

Inspiration is where you find it. Be the lighthouse and inspire the entire world to create peace in our time.

The eagle understands, it *feels* the wind. What a thing! To be so in tune with one's body to be able to move without moving!

Wahe Guru!

The eagle knows—let go, free your mind and soar like the eagle.

The magic is contagious, open your heart and together we'll heal the world.

Bless you, Sat Nam.

Hope for the future

Whether it's hope or inspiration that drives you to keep pushing yourself up off the floor, be the lighthouse and see it done.

The power of God lies within you. "*Ong Namo Guru Dev Namo*," puts it right there in your hands.

Even when you're all alone in the still of the night, know that you are God and so is everyone and everything else.

You are God and no one can ever take that away from you. It's the greatest secret ever told. God is all encompassing, the all that is, all knowing and all pervasive, everywhere.

There is no thing that is not God, help the world to remember, bring hope to those who have none, shine so bright that the next ten thousand generations will see your light.

Be the light to guide their way on.

Bless you God and thank you.

Sat Nam.

Faith

Surfing along, riding the waves of life, the ups and downs I encounter along the way, I realized that life is nothing more than a series of interconnected adventures. Everything affects everything else. Every deed, word, thought or action directly affects the rest of my life.

Life itself is a meditation and many things exist to pull you off your center. Challenges that come up along the way, adversity that seeks to drag you into despair.

It's as easy as you make it.

The demons get bigger, but so too does your sword and shield. Know that they are there, use the tools you've been given and you can overcome any obstacle.

Whether you call them demons or by some other metaphor, those challenges exist in every life. It's how we face them that shapes our life and our future.

I know personally, when I'm too busy chasing about, trying to create profit, that I don't write. I don't like what I become when that happens.

Sinking into despair isn't an option, despite the money demons best efforts.

The money will come, everything's in place, even though I can't consciously see it. Have faith, and vanquish those demons.

Sat Nam.

Dragon slaying

I'm going dragon slaying, who's with me?

Call it what you will, but everyone has their own obstacles to overcome.

Love knows no limits, nor does God, open your heart and allow yourself to be God. Let the love flow freely, hold no limits.

Let go.

Let go.

Let go and let God through.

At times I feel lost, I have no money coming in and yet my heart's greatest desire is to help people.

I've achieved no financial gain this day, yet I feel it has already been one of my most productive ever.

I realized recently that I'd rather wander the Earth barefoot and penniless than go back to my old life. It may yet come to that, but I don't think so.

You see, I have the inside track. A very dear friend gifted me with a magic flashlight that I shine into the dark corners of my mind when fear and doubt begin to creep in.

They know not of their importance, yet they're a lighthouse nevertheless.

Honor the God in yourself and in all that you see and the rest will take care of itself.

Peace be with you my friends. Shine on into the night. Now come on, sit down and let's do some yoga together.

Pains and trains

Often, our greatest pain can bring about our greatest growth, if we but step aside and let it happen.

It's easy to say there's more to life than money, but to live it, now that can be another matter entirely.

I realized, just now, how much of my existence I've spent either worrying about money or trying to acquire it. Right now it seems like all I was doing was chasing my tail as I ran around in one big circle. I'd like to think I've come full circle.

The abundance train's coming my way, though this morning it felt like it had derailed along the way.

It doesn't really matter which way it goes, this is the year of change after all.

Hold no attachments, not to potential outcomes, nor to persons, places, or things. Everything is about to change anyway. And just when you think you've got it all figured out, everything will change again. Life's not about trying to wrap your head around everything.

Allow yourself to be God. Forget everything, and allow it to come through.

Life isn't about money, accept the fact that you are God and allow it to happen.

Your success is already guaranteed, so in the meantime, come on, let's do some yoga together. Sit down and we'll tune in...

"Ong Namo Guru Dev Namo."

Water

*T*o be blessed with such abundance, to possess water in sufficient quantity to freely splash it upon our bodies, to be able to drink at will, to have so much when so many have none.

Yes, I know it's heavy. Come on, I'll help you.

Believe in yourself, I do, as does God.

I left my job, taking it on faith that the universe would provide for me.

To hold water in my hands and let it fall freely upon my tongue, at last I understand the true nature of wealth.

In these times when so many have so little, take nothing for granted.

If a single bottle of water contains that much magic, imagine what the rest of life holds in store for you!

Wahe Guru!

Water II

*D*ecember the 1st, 2005.

It was today that I discovered one of life's greatest pleasures, that of cool water splashing upon my tongue. To freely drink of clean water, I know I am a wealthy man indeed!

This has indeed been the year of change, 2005 has. Nothing will ever be the same again, not for me, not for you, not for the world.

Change is a good thing though, if we embrace rather than resist it.

I'm just the messenger, the guy with the bucket of water.

There's more than enough to go around. You have to want to drink, you have to be willing to do the work. Are you?

I fall down, a lot sometimes, but every time I do, my angel picks me up, dusts me off and wraps me in her golden wings.

I'll see her again soon. Not high in the mountains above the desert, but someplace new this time, along the shore….

I cannot do it for you, you have to push yourself up off the floor, but I'll be right there beside you every step of the way, my brothers, my sisters.

Now come on, let's do some yoga together.

72 Percent

I had a dream last night, 72 Percent, 3 points short, failure….

Does it mean anything? Was it "just" a dream? Whatever it was, it just is.

No attachments means no attachments to a n y t h i n g, be it a person, place, thing, outcome or desire.

I asked for it, though I would never have known what I was getting myself into. Not that I would do anything differently, but oh what I got myself into! Wahe Guru!

I've been through the shadow of the valley of death. I've seen hell on Earth and across the ages I've seen more suffering and lost more friends than I care to recount. All of this, from fear and separateness.

It's time to end all of that right now.

If you remember nothing else from this book, make it these three words, I am God.

Repeat after me, "I am God… I am God… I am God."

Carry it with you in your heart, now and for all time, and together we'll heal the world.

That's what being a lighthouse is all about, being a messenger of hope and peace in these dark times we walk through. Pain and suffering abound, rise above it and together we'll heal the world, three little words that will free us all, "I am God."

Stop chasing about and spread the light.

It all starts with knowing and feeling those three little words down to the core of your being.

I am God…

I am God…

I am God and so is everyone and everything else.

Sat Nam.

Birth

I was born on a yoga mat, high in the desert. I realized just now, that's my home, a yoga mat.

Everything is transitory, even the mat itself.

If nothing else, I can shout from the highest mountain, "I am a teacher!"

What will you proclaim?

It's okay, you have plenty of time to think about it. Come on, I'll climb with you.

We can chant along the way… do you know the words to the Ray Man Shabad?

Come on, I'll teach you….

Commitment

*T*he greatest commitment, a thousand days of Bound Lotus, 80 down, only 920 to go.

Now if I could just get paid for it, doing/teaching yoga that is.

The abundance train appears to have derailed on its way to my house. Maybe it went past on a day I slept in….

What now God?

I actually asked that, out loud, over a dozen times tonight, as I realized that chasing about trying to create profit costs me two ways. It actually costs me money, trying to create profit, and what's worse, when I'm chasing about I don't write.

The writing itself has long since become a meditation for me.

Considering how much money's gone out and how little's come in, I was very calm about it. I just kept asking, what now God? Over and over again, maybe even two dozen times….

Am I to sell everything I own? Then what?

I even redecorated part of the house, with no money coming in, why? I've spent all this money, all of it on nice but very little of it necessary things. What am I doing?

Chasing about….

Where is the abundance? We're about at the end of the money, I don't really want to go back to corporate America….

What now God?

Just sitting at home doing yoga all day long isn't the answer. Something is though….

Then there's the matter of this cold that won't go away. I know the two are somehow tied together, I've been too busy chasing about to see the answer….

What now God? What's the answer? How do I help people and earn a living at the same time? How do I tie the two together? What of my writing?

Winter Solstice approaches… it was Summer Solstice that led us down this path, to career change and that of being a lighthouse. I know I need the three days of Tantric….

I know the abundance is coming, but it really can't take much longer, I'm about at the end of the money. What now God?

Guide my hand so that I may be the lighthouse. Give me the strength to carry the water to those who have none. Help me to shine out into the darkness to guide their way on, help me to help heal the world. Help me to see my own hand in front of my face, help me to find my way to abundance.

Bless you and thank you God, for always being there for me, for answering all of my prayers and providing for all of my needs before I even know I have them.

Bless you, Sat Nam.

I lay awake

*T*he house creaks, it too is unable to sleep.

I didn't really put any planning into this. I had some money so I quit my job to become a yoga teacher. Now the money's almost gone, and how much effort have I put into that?

Right now it seems like I've chased about a lot....

What now God, what's the answer? What do I do now!?

"Simple, be the lighthouse."

How do I do that and earn money?

I need your help God. It's my hearts greatest desire to help people, help me make that happen. Guide my way on....

Come, everyone, and bath in the light with me. We'll get there together, I promise, you have but to put forth the effort. Now let's tune in and do some yoga.

"Ong Namo Guru Dev Namo."

Open your eyes

*I*t's amazing how the briefest of hellos from the dearest of friends can lift ones spirits.

In this case, my Bound Lotus mentor, a lighthouse if ever there was one.

Day 80, today will be 81, the deepest commitment I've ever made.

I've never been married, but this is something similar but far deeper, the union of me with my soul, in this Bound Lotus, this thing I've come to love and respect as surrender pose.

It's time, come on....

Yoga will save the world, come, it starts with you, right now, on your mat, wherever you are. Free your mind and free the world.

Inspiration is all around you, open your eyes....

Where did the magic go?

*R*emember the magic of childhood?

Why did you grow up?

Was it because of responsibility or dedication to duty?

Remember the splendor you once viewed everything with?

For me that magic was *Star Wars*, how about you?

Thanks to Kundalini Yoga, I live in the magic. You can too, it's as easy as Ong Namo Guru Dev Namo.

Celebrate the light

*W*inter Solstice approaches, and with it, three more days of White Tantric Yoga.

This Kundalini Yoga truly is a sacred science if ever there was one!

Friends old and new, my brothers and sisters from across the globe will gather in celebration of the light, to be the lighthouse, to help humanity usher in the coming Age of Aquarius.

The time is nigh, to rise to the challenge or be crushed beneath it.

Seven years may seem like a long time, but it'll be here before you know it.

Everything will change, come, let's get ready for it….

Sit down here with me and let's all surrender together. I can do it and I know you can too.

You get out of it what you put into it. Put forth your best effort and the universe will support you, God will support you and I will support you from now until the end of time.

Remember those five little words, that's the key to it all, how it all begins....

"*Ong Namo Guru Dev Namo.*"

Living in the light

See the light, be the light, be the lighthouse.

Where do we go from here God?

"*Into the light.*"

Could you be a little more specific please?

"*You mean like turn left at the next light?*"

Yeah, that'd be good.

"*Seeking the path to letting go is something else to let go of. It's not about calculating what two plus two equals, but rather about being the answer. All of the thinking and seeking keeps you from being. Cease all of the chasing about, the worrying and trying to wrap your head around everything. Your success is assured, let go and let it happen.*"

Sigh.

Ong Namo Guru Dev Namo.

"*Excellent. Shuniya. Relax, let go and be the answer. Become the light, be the lighthouse. Sat Nam.*"

Ong Namo Guru Dev Namo.

Ong Namo Guru Dev Namo.

Remember to laugh and allow yourself to cry.

Come, sit, let's do some yoga and together we'll ride the wave of light into the coming Age of Aquarius.

Bless you, Sat Nam.

You are the lighthouse

*U*nplug and hear the universe, it speaks to you. God speaks to everyone all the time, who listens?

Plot your course, you are the captain, you are the lighthouse.

Wahe Guru!

It is *your* life, never give away your free will. Live life to the fullest and achieve your highest potential, that of being the lighthouse, and being God.

You are the lighthouse.

You are the lighthouse.

You are the lighthouse.

Forgive yourself and everyone else, free your mind and allow yourself to be God.

Sat Nam.

God's love

*P*rosperity and abundance will rain down upon you if you but allow it to happen.

Open yourself to God's love and allow it to flow freely though you. Be the lighthouse, be the conduit of love and light that you were born to be, show the universe that **you are the lighthouse!**

Plant your feet squarely, stand tall, square your shoulders and repeat after me, I am the lighthouse.

Shout from the highest mountain to the lowest valley, I am the lighthouse!

Let no stone go unturned in your quest. God is everywhere, under every rock no matter how large or how small.

Repeat it with me.

I am the lighthouse.

I am the lighthouse.

I am the lighthouse.

Now and for all time, you are the lighthouse. May you shine bright for all of your days and nights.

Sat Nam.

Shine on

*B*ound Lotus, Day 89.

On this the eve of my leaving for Winter Solstice, many things at last become clear.

I can see and feel prosperity and abundance approaching. The worries have all drifted away on the breeze, spirited away by my friend and partner in creation—God.

Wahe Guru!

There is but one way to describe the complete surrender that Bound Lotus has brought about in me—Wahe Guru!

Wahe Guru—*I am in ecstasy when I experience the Indescribable Wisdom.*

The year of change comes to a close and it's time to shine.

Shed your fears, your inhibitions, your attachments and all things that no longer serve you, and be the light. You are the lighthouse, it's time to shine.

You have the energy and the strength of God within you. It's time to let it all out, *you are God*, shine on through the days and nights to come.

Shine on and be the lighthouse.

Sat Nam.

God's messenger

*G*od's messenger, Yogi Bhajan....

Times change, things change, people change and move on, even angels, it's an inevitable part of life. You can't stop the change and no amount of wanting can make it otherwise.

Thank you Yogi Bhajan for the gift of this Kundalini Yoga, thank you God for giving us the tools to let go.

No attachments to anything, not even to angels....

Let go, surrender to the nothingness, the stillness, and awaken to your higher consciousness. Become an empty vessel to be filled with love and light.

It's as easy as you make it….

Trees and angels

So much of the world is completely unaware of the true nature of our existence on this plane. Be the lighthouse and show them the way.

So much hustling and bustling, scurrying to and fro, where does it all lead? Not to shuniya that's for certain.

My angel moved on, so many others in need….

In exchange, God gifted me with the most magnificent of trees. I wish my dad were here to tell me what kind of tree it was….

Its Spanish moss blows in the breeze as it stands amongst its brothers and sisters, standing across the ages….

Inspiration is all around you, you have but to open your eyes….

Thank you God

Thank you God for granting me the courage to see me through what is to come.

Thank you God for granting me the strength to be the lighthouse.

Thank you God for the gift of this Kundalini Yoga, the means of my awakening.

Thank you God for helping me to be the lighthouse.

Bless you God.

Sat Nam.

Footprints in the sand

I realized, this has become a journal of my life. You have but to read in between the footprints to see where I've been.

Even shuniya is a choice, zero, nothing. You don't need the solitude of a remote mountaintop to find quiet. With practice you can filter out any amount of noise.

Enter into the stillness, become one with it and make it your own.

The light will guide you, but ultimately you have to find your own way up the mountain.

You have to do the work, no one can do it for you.

What are you waiting for?

Let it flow

*S*at Nam—truth is my identity.

I am the lighthouse and so are you.

Who are you and where are you going with your life?

Sat Nam, you are the lighthouse, make it your truth.

Anything is possible, never allow limited thinking to hold you back. All things are possible if you have the determination and apply yourself.

Take Mount Everest, many tried and failed to climb to the top of the world until someone **did** it.

Certainty of purpose—doing God's work—guarantees your success even if you don't see it.

Be the lighthouse, carry the water and be about your father's work.

Sat Nam.

Do

*D*o.

Do.

Do.

Be in the flow and do.

Do everything with all of your heart. Pour all of your love into all that you do.

Do for others, selflessly. Neither expect nor want anything in return, simply be the lighthouse.

Share in all that you have and all that you are.

Do.

Do.

Do.

Don't think about it, don't write about it, don't talk about it, just do it.

You are the lighthouse.

Sat Nam.

31 minutes

How long is 31 minutes?

Bound into the symbol for Infinity, it seems an eternity. Then again, time doesn't really exist. It's just a blink of the eye....

Everything fades as you merge with the Infinite. Surrender to it. Want nothing for yourself, ask for nothing for yourself, surrender and be the lighthouse.

Be the light

May all of your days be filled with sunshine, and your nights with warmth, may the light guide your way on.

Chant with all of your heart, God's listening.

Ong Namo Guru Dev Namo.

Feel it vibrate through your soul, live it, be it.

I am God, I am the lighthouse.

Repeat it with me, I am God, I am the lighthouse.

I am God, I am the lighthouse.

I am God, I am the lighthouse.

Feel it, live it, be it, be the light.

Sat Nam

You have to earn it

Bound Lotus gives you pain before it takes it away.

Bald eagles came to the lake to do some White Tantric Yoga with us. They soared high above us, as if to say, "Let go, fly like us!"

And fly we did!

The body isn't real, so how then can the pain be real? What body?

The pain will go away, but you have to earn it.

I'm just a guy, the guy with the bucket of water.

I am immortal and so are you.

Undying, the eternal all that is.

I am God and so are you.

I am immortal and so are you.

Appearances change and one day I'll leave this physical body behind, but I am I immortal and so are you.

Sat Nam.

Dreams fade

*T*hings change, times change. Old friends leave, new ones come.

I spent Christmas Eve with a bald eagle, soaring above the lake, free....

It's your life, what are you doing with it?

It's your garbage pit, how fast are you going to empty it?

Not even the sky's the limit if you're willing to do the work.

Freedom will come if you allow it.

Surrender and live in the now, live in the flow and be the lighthouse.

Sat Nam.

Christmas Eve

*F*lames dance as the sparks drift high into the night sky.

Christmas Eve, round the campfire....

Where are you, where are you going?

Dances with eagles

Eagles came, to guide my way home, to guide me to be the lighthouse.

Clarity, sureness of purpose and a quiet stillness are my constant companions, the aftereffects of three days of White Tantric Yoga. How long it stays is entirely up to me....

A great many things come to light, the effect of doing the equivalent of years of yoga in just three days... three days by the lake dancing with eagles....

You have that power within you, the power to let it go all in an instant, be free and soar like the eagle. Spread your wings and be the lighthouse.

Now let's do some yoga together....

Day 100

Bound Lotus, Day 100... who would ever have imagined such a thing....

The feeling is indescribable, not even Wahe Guru seems adequate.

Walking with angels, flying with eagles as I surrender to the realization that I am not my body, now that is Bound Lotus in a nutshell.

Of course, part of the experience comes from chanting the Ray Man Shabad as I surrender....

Unplugging, awakening, to my divine essence, that is what Bound Lotus is, and all after only 100 days! Imagine what the next 100 will be like! Wahe Guru!

Dividends

*Y*ou don't have to be flexible to do Bound Lotus or even any form of yoga/meditation. You'll become flexible through regular practice.

You get out what you put into it....

You're earning dividends for yourself, freeing your mind and healing your soul in the process of letting go.

It's as easy as Ong Namo Guru Dev Namo, let's tune in and do some yoga together.

Into the mist

*T*he year of change draws to a close... 2005, nothing will ever be the same again, least of all me!

Wahe Guru! What a ride it's been! Who would ever have dreamt this was where my life was leading me? Certainly not me, that's for sure!

Into the mist of 2006 we go, writing our own future in the days and weeks to come. Turn the page and see where it leads....

It's your life, create what you will. Put pen to paper and write your life, it's all there for the choosing....

I stand at the crossroads, unable to see a clear path before my feet, yet I know my path. How can that be my destiny? I'm just a guy....

"You chose that path for yourself long before you were ever born into this life."

That doesn't make it any easier....

"The sands of life are ever drifting, the wind ever shifting, move with it, and through it grow into the realization that you are God. You cannot escape it, open your eyes and fulfill the destiny you have chosen for yourself. Do not let fear of the unknown cloud your judgment or forestall your choices. You know what must be done, for the good of all. Yes, there will be sacrifices, but what's more important, conquering the mind and being the lighthouse or being a slave to your ego? I will be with you, every step of the way, to guide you through the mist. Step into the role you have chosen for yourself, it's time to begin the next phase of your life."

Time to wake the children

What do you see when you look out the window? The wind blowing through the trees or a world so caught up in its own goings on that it's destroying itself? Or even both, as the wind's eternal....

It's time to wake the children.

Many yearn for a better world, one of peace, abundance and friendship, a world without war....

The New Year dawns, and I catch myself caught up in the game, distracted, doing this and doing that rather than relaxing and being in the flow... it's easy to do if you unplug.

It's all just a game, you don't win or lose, *you live*. How you live is entirely up to you. You can float between the stars if you choose.

I chose to be the lighthouse, you?

Seekers

We're all seekers of one thing or another, what is it that you're seeking?

Truth?

Love?

Peace?

Light?

All of the above?

What is it that guides your way on?

What is the driving force in your life?

What is it that motivates you?

What is it that gives you cause to do the things that you do?

Selfless desire to serve others?

To be the lighthouse and help heal the world?

To find peace in our time?

What gives you pause to think, in the still of the night?

Drift into the wind, enter into the river of life and become the answer.

Sat Nam.

God's breath

Bound Lotus is God's breath in your lungs, it's God's blessing upon your soul.

Chant and God chants with you.

Bound into the symbol for Infinity, chanting the Ray Man Shabad, I can feel it healing my soul across all time and space. It's proof, to me, that I am not my body, that we are timeless, and that we are all God's children.

The pain will come, surrender and it will go away, which is why I sometimes refer to it as surrender pose. The mind rails, wanting out. Surrender your mind, body and soul to the posture, chant with all your heart, free your mind and be the lighthouse.

Sat Nam.

I'll watch over you

Relax, stretch out and let go of your body. I'll watch over you....

Enter into the silence and hear the universe vibrate.

Tune out all of the mindless chatter and hear the indescribable song, feel its gentle caress upon your soul, feel its soothing touch guiding your way back to the light.

Feel it guiding your way through the night.

Feel it in the depths of your soul and know that you are God.

Sat Nam.

Day 108

*B*ound Lotus, Day 108.

"Try 31," she said, Mahan Kirn that is, 31 minutes of Bound Lotus. To some that might sound like, "Walk to the moon." But what she gifted me with was an invitation to see God's face in the mirror and fly among the stars, to lift out of my body and to experience the divine firsthand.

It was an invitation to hold the sun in my hands, to dance with angels as they chant,

> *"Ray man eh bidh jog kamaa-o*
> *Singee saach akapat kanthalaa*
> *Dhi-aan bibhoot charaa-o*
> *Taatee geho aatam bas kar kee*
> *Bhicchhaa naam adhaarang*
> *Baajay param taar tat har ko*
> *Upajai raag rasaarang*
> *Ughatai taan tarang rang*
> *At gi-aan geet bandhaanang*
> *Chak chak rehay dayv daanav mun*
> *Chhak chhak bayom bivaanang*
> *Aatam upadays bhays sanjam ko*
> *Jaap so ajapaa jaapai*
> *Sadaa rehai kanchan see kaayaa*
> *Kaal na kabahoo bayaapai."*

It was all of that and so much more, Gods loving touch upon my face, a ride on a star, an invitation to become the eternal light, to be the lighthouse....

Sat Nam, and thank you Mahan Kirn Kaur Khalsa.

Angels at your side

A ngels can't do Bound Lotus, White Tantric Yoga, Kundalini Yoga or any other form of yoga for that matter. They don't have bodies....

They are ever at your side as you surrender to the posture, offering support and chanting along with you as they shower you with love, light and energy.

It is only now that I begin to comprehend the magic of what this is, this creation you hold in your hands. It's evolved, as have I, through regular practice.

Today was my 108th day of Bound Lotus, 108, the number for Infinity, exactly how long I plan to practice.

This morning as I folded myself up, during the ambrosial hours of the amrit vela, I could feel the angels at my side. Their hearts yearn to experience such things, something only we are capable of. They watch, fascinated with the process of our evolution.

The pain was unimaginable, but there they were, whispering in my ear, "*You can do it.*"

Tomorrow is to be 31 minutes, the penultimate goal, a sacred objective if ever there was one. I wonder what it will be like... only one way to find out!

Whatever your regular practice might be, keep at it and know that angels are ever at your side.

Sat Nam.

I met God

*J*anuary 5th, 2006, Bound Lotus, Day 109.

So, what was 31 minutes like, you ask?

I met God.

No metaphors or analogies, no frame of reference or comparison. I met God.

Each day brings a new experience, suffice it to say, Bound Lotus is my path to God.

Today we sat down together as I surrendered, we chanted together and even relaxed together afterwards.

From this moment forward everything I will ever do will be easy compared to 31 minutes of Bound Lotus. It puts everything in perspective.

I won't sugar coat it for you, Bound Lotus is the most difficult kriya in all of yoga. At times the pain is almost unbearable, the mind ready to explode. Holding it for 31 minutes is every bit as challenging as White Tantric Yoga, if not more so.

Breath, and chant with all your heart, still your mind and body, relax into it and enjoy the experience. Sit back and enjoy the ride!

To be blessed with the ability to do such a thing! Wahe Guru!

Time stood still, I met God.

Every day there will be less pain, and eventually none at all, until then my friends.

Sat Nam.

You can do it

*T*he pain is mind numbingly intense as the body seemingly tears itself apart from the inside.

The universe whispers in my ear, "*You can do it*," and I do it, hold the posture for 31 minutes.

Nothing is impossible, 31 minutes of Bound Lotus is living proof.

It is a doorway, a gateway to God, a portal to universal understanding.

Maybe I'm only on the first step, but I'll keep on climbing.

Whatever your path, keep on climbing your mountain, your own way back to God.

Sat Nam.

Anticipation

*T*he face tingles in anticipation of the coming light. Sit, listen....

Do you hear it?

Relax and hear, enter into the stillness and become it. Shuniya, zero....

Blank and receptive, the universe speaks to you.

Feel it vibrate within you as you become.

With your every thought and action, be consciously aware of that which you are creating.

Still yourself, feel it within you, make it your own and become the stillness.

What do you hear? Everything and yet nothing at the same time?

Peace….

Feel the beating of your heart, the blood coursing through your body, your very own universe, energy pouring through you as you become the lighthouse.

You are the light, eternal and undying.

Now let's do some yoga together!

Stories to share

Scribbles, words on a page, things that come to me. I write them down to share….

This is my journey through Kundalini Yoga, my path. And yes, Bound Lotus is my ticket home, but that doesn't mean it's yours.

It is most assuredly not a beginner's set and it is without question the most difficult kriya in all of yoga. My unbridled enthusiasm for it aside, it took years of doing yoga before I even learned of it, let alone was ready to attempt the posture.

And it hurts too, mentally as well as physically. The pain fades with time though, and one day there'll be none. Until that day….

Whether or not you can do it or not doesn't matter. Within Kundalini Yoga there are thousands of other postures, meditations, and yoga sets. Any one of them might bring you experiences far beyond my own. Enjoy the finding out!

That's where it all begins, how that doorway to the divine eases open, ever so slowly, with time and effort.

This is the story of my journey, come, sit by the fire and share your story.

Sat Nam.

Reach for it

*F*reedom is within your grasp, reach for it with both hands.

It's an investment in yourself, how hard are you willing to work for it?

What would you give up to free your mind?

Everything?

Some things?

Nothing?

I'll stand watch

*S*leep my child, you're safe here, nestled in your angel's warm blanket of light, wrapped in God's arms.

Let go of your tension, all your worries, I'll stand watch this night. Be at peace my dear child.

Slip into nothingness, fade into the wind and let your breath carry you back to the light.

Sat Nam.

While the world sleeps

*R*ise up, while the world sleeps. Do it for yourself.

Smile and see the reaction it brings, see God's face reflected back.

Rise up, while the world sleeps. Sadhana, an investment in yourself.

Rise up in the angel's mist, the predawn, and invest in your soul.

Come, meditate, chant and do some yoga with us, do it for yourself while the world sleeps. An investment with a tenfold return....

Rise up, and the rest is easy.

What is freedom worth? How hard are you willing to work to free your mind and heal your soul?

Sat Nam.

Walk with God

*S*at Nam, what is your truth?

You have in your hands, an invitation from God, to find your truth, to find your way home, to be the lighthouse and so much more. What will you do with it?

The universe beckons, what will you do?

Feel the Earth through bare feet, walk free through grass, sand and water. Feel the fresh air upon your face, the wind at your back.

Walk with God at your side, among the stars, and hold the universe in your hands.

Sat Nam.

The universe is calling

*R*ay Man eh, Sat Nam.

Oh my mind, truth is my identity.

What is your truth, your identity?

No more chasing about, allow the Ray Man Shabad to flow through you and wash over you as you surrender. Quit seeking them and life's mysteries will reveal themselves to you. Empty your mind and hear the universe calling.

Ray Man eh, Sat Nam.

Ray Man eh, Sat Nam.

Ray Man eh, Sat Nam.

What is your truth, your identity?

The universe is calling.

Answer the call.

Sat Nam.

Open the door

*K*nock, knock.

God's at the door, who will answer?

Open the door, let yourself in. Don't make yourself wait out in the cold. That's what separateness does, creates enemies and animosity, spreads fear and dissent among us, keeps us from being God.

We're all one being. Until everyone lives that truth we'll continue to have pain and suffering in the world.

Open the door and let yourself in.

It's cold outside....

Spring approaches

Soon the grass will grow tall, the air filled with the sound of children laughing and playing, free of the cares of adults.

The sun will reach high and warm our days as the light pushes the darkness away.

Leaves and snow will come and go.

Light fades, temperatures fall as the cycle of life begins anew.

Spring approaches....

Priorities

Distractions come, to pull you from the path, the road to shuniya.

In the stillness, the silence, you will see them for what they are.

Relax into the silence, still yourself and be.

No more chasing distractions, prioritize.

Kundalini Yoga is for everyone, everywhere. Even just a few minutes a day....

Focus on what's important. Chasing about or reconnecting with the Infinite?

Yes, in the modern world we have daily tasks, perform them with grace and purity. Make your every step a meditation, be it earning an income or carrying the water to those who have none, do it with all your heart and be the lighthouse.

All things will come to you when you no longer seek or want them. Detachment is the key, be still, in the silence. Focus on the things that really matter, learn from what you have experienced. Feel and be.

Now let's do some yoga.

Footsteps in the night

The silence echoes to Infinity.

The mind is the key, the gateway to understanding.

Free your mind and hold the world in your hands, heal the world with your light.

Live in the light and know that you are God.

Sat Nam, this is where it all begins.

Dwell in God and free your mind.

Come back to the light, now and for all time.

Angels will catch you should you fall.

Relax and hear the rain on the roof, remember the magic and be the light.

Sat Nam.

Into the light

*T*he pain fades as the light within grows, how's that for incentive?

Every day there's less pain, I know one day there'll be none. Until that day, keep working.

Saying the body isn't real is one thing, definitive detachment, now that's something entirely different.

It hurts, I know it does, but today there was less pain than yesterday and less than the day before.

You get out of it what you put into it, surrendering to the posture brings pain, but is the pain real or is it all in your mind?

Obviously, don't hurt yourself, but also challenge yourself.

The pain fades as the energy flows through you, calm your body and mind, breathe, chant, and feel alive with the love and light of the universe! Wahe Guru!

All there is to it is to do it.

Where we go from here is anyone's guess, I'm going into the light, who's with me?

Shine on through the night

*A*live and free, what else is there?

Free of pain and living in the light, the answers come, all needs are met. Serve and help others where you can.

See others not as others but an extension of the self, yet another part of the eternal and undying God, the all that is.

God cannot be harmed, if everyone knew such things, war would not exist for why would anyone seek to destroy the indestructible?

Show them the way, share the warmth and light you have been blessed with.

See the magic in all things, smile and the universe smiles with you.

Have faith, in yourself and in God and shine on through the night.

Sat Nam.

The beginning

*T*his is only the beginning, the journey never ends.

Life is a blank page to be filled with experience. Ups and downs yes, but learn from the process and enjoy it!

What will you create with your page? Will you share your page with the world, giving pieces to those who have none?

What of the children, they are the future. What world would you have them inherit? One filled with peace and joy? Be the lighthouse and together we'll make it happen.

Now we could go on about being the lighthouse and keep talking about yoga, but let's **do** some yoga. Yoga is going to heal the world. It's a practical tool that everyone can apply to their lives.

See to it that the world no longer needs guns, we could make yoga mats instead!

Now let's tune in....

Desire

*T*eaching propels the desire to learn, feel the interplay between your body and the Infinite.

Your heartbeat is that of the universe itself, seeking a better understanding of itself, creating experience during a journey of self discovery. Where that journey goes from here is entirely up to you.

The mind is yours to master if you have the will. Kundalini Yoga is the way.

Meditate unto the Infinite, transcend the body and propel yourself beyond space and time.

It all starts with Ong Namo Guru Dev Namo, five little words on the path to self discovery….

Friendship

*V*ery often in life, the greatest gifts we ever receive are the immaterial ones, like friendship.

A dear friend, someone to guide you when you have lost your way, one who sits up all night with you when you are sick, or just to laugh till dawn.

Ever at your side, they will get up at 3 am to do sadhana with you, or even climb the highest mountain just to enjoy your company. Treasure them, always.

Sat Nam.

Choose and act

*E*ven in the dark, the light is always there, and yes, the darkness is there even in the light. It's all about perception. What do you see? Neither holds sway over the other, but rather they form a symbiotic relationship. You can't have one without the other.

The light fades as the sun sets, just as the darkness retreats with the rising of the sun, all part of the cycle of life.

Yes the light comes and goes, but you carry that same energy within you, you are your own sun, with your own connection to the universe. What will you do with it?

I'm just the messenger, I can help guide your way, but ultimately you have to make the choice and do the work yourself. Yes, I can point the way, but the path is yours to take, or not. Paths change and evolve, so too it is with choices.

You have but to choose and act.

Sat Nam.

Choices

*T*he choices we make directly affect our path and our lives. Several months ago I chose to be the lighthouse, and yes, I do a lot of yoga in between teaching and writing.

No matter what your schedule, there's time to do some yoga, some meditation.

How much effort are you willing to put forth to free your mind, to reconnect with the divine, to become the stillness and be God?

The choice is yours, it's as easy as you make it....

So what will it be?

The trees stripped bare

*O*nce proud limbs reduced to stubs....

Why?

Why does war exist? You can't kill God, why try?

Why make war on yourself? Why harm yourself? Why take from yourself?

Not everyone remembers that we are all a part of God, be the lighthouse and help them to remember.

Sat Nam.

Dreams

*A*t last we reach the point where it all takes definitive shape, the moment we can point to a date on a calendar and say, "There, that is when it will happen."

No more blindly stumbling about in the dark, no more pursuit, of anything.

If 2005 was the year of change, 2006 is the year of awakening.

Awaken to the reality that you are the lighthouse, and that you are God.

It's time we as a race truly find ourselves and walk among the stars. You can help make that happen, we've been lost long enough.

Be the lighthouse and help the world to find themselves.

Things take shape, and dreams do come true if you let them.

Be the lighthouse and see to it that everyone can follow their dreams.

Sat Nam.

Just like that

*M*iracles happen just like that if you put in the effort and have faith in the universe.

All your dreams can come true just like that if you're willing to carry the water and be the lighthouse.

Just like that.

Be the instrument of change, be the fulcrum the entire universe turns on.

Hold God in your hands and just like that, anything can happen.

Sat Nam.

How far

*I*t's amazing how one sentence can be so profound and spark so much thought.

A one line message from the dearest of friends, "that's right, that's the way it works...you put the effort in and God has to do 10x the work!"

Ten times the work! Wahe Guru!

If God will do ten times the work, how hard will **you** work? How much effort will you put into freeing your mind and becoming the lighthouse? How far will you carry the bucket of water?

How far?

My path

*T*here's always new ground to cover, new territory to explore.

Ideas flow when you are clear, the mind empty. What you do with them is entirely up to you.

So many things crystallize in the stillness, empty your mind and discover them.

Feel the pulsing of your heart with every fiber of your being. Turn the corner and let go, master the mind and free yourself from your ego.

Be still, and listen, hear the universe calling, guiding your way home.

Every path is as unique as the individual, like snowflakes, no two are alike.

Open your mind, and your heart, and find your way home.

My path, my journey, is through Kundalini Yoga, you?

Turn the handle

*T*he silence deepens as you move into it. How far does it go?

Let's find out....

The greatest adventure of all, into the mind and discovering God within! Wahe Guru!

The sun sets on another day, darkness edges in. Soon the stars will follow.

Your heart pulses in rhythm with the vibration of the universe, tune in and feel the Infinite all around you.

The final doorway... turn the handle and be pulled out into the vacuum. Free....

Turn the handle....

Turn the handle and live free, one with the Infinite, one with God.

Turn the handle....

How simple it is

*B*ecome so still you can hear the snow fall....

It's too warm... the snow returns to whence it came, melting, merging with the Infinite. How simple it is....

If it's cold enough, it stays snow, too warm, it turns back into water. How simple it is....

Open your senses and be the stillness.

Tingle with awareness and be truth.

Sat Nam—*truth is my identity*.

Relax and feel truth vibrate through you, relax and be.

Ang Sang Wahe Guru

*S*tray thoughts come, let them pass through you.

A great many things will try your patience if given the chance.

Ang Sang Wahe Guru—*God is with my every limb, every millimeter, every situation of mine*.

What else is there to say?

Ang Sang Wahe Guru.

See God in all things, live, and feel God within you, Ang Sang Wahe Guru, you are God, you are the lighthouse.

Sat Nam.

Be present

*T*ake your every breath consciously, full and deep, ever mindful of what your thoughts and actions are creating.

Be aware, not mindless.

It's your mind, who's in charge, you or it? It's how you react to things, that's what's important.

Yes, we have to clean the house, do laundry, go to the store, cook, but do all of those things consciously. Sometime when you're cleaning the house, try chanting and see how divine of an experience it is! Wahe Guru!

Everything can be a meditation, from splitting firewood to washing dishes, carrying a bucket of water or even writing about your journey....

It's what you make it, life is, how you live each moment that defines who and what you are as a person. What will you do with it?

How far will you carry that bucket of water?

Free your mind and be God. Be present and be God.

Sat Nam.

Stray thoughts come

A great many things will try your patience if given the chance.

Stray thoughts come, let them pass through you.

Move beyond the mind, the body, pain, even time itself. Let the stillness wash over you as you merge with the Infinite and reunite your soul with God.

Drink creativity with every inhalation, exhale all pain and fear. Be love and be the light that shines through the night.

Sat Nam.

A reminder

I'll keep saying it until the whole world is free, until everyone awakens to their true nature and becomes the lighthouse.

Be the lighthouse.

Free your mind, fly with angels and eagles, be the lighthouse.

You are the eternal light, shine bright and be the lighthouse.

Take that leap of faith, let go of everything and be the lighthouse my sisters and brothers.

Within Kundalini Yoga are a nearly endless number of tools to facilitate said letting go, avail yourself of them and be the lighthouse.

Be the lighthouse and see to it that there are no more killing fields from now until the end of time.

Be the lighthouse.

Be the lighthouse.

Be the lighthouse.

Sat Nam.

How far indeed

*Y*ou have the bucket of water, spiritual knowledge, how far will you carry it to those who have none, to those in need, to those who seek the light yet know not where to look?

How far indeed?

Gifts such as these are to be shared with the universe.

Ek Ong Kar Sat Nam Siri Wahe Guru—*The Creator and all creation are one. This is our True Identity. The ecstasy of this wisdom is Great beyond words.*

How far will you carry the water so that YOU may drink?

How far?

How far indeed?

Be the key

*F*ree your mind and free yourself from all pain.

Banish the demons, those things that serve only to pull you off center, away from shuniya, and experience ecstasy beyond description.

Doubt evaporates, replaced with an undeniable certainty of purpose.

The path is clear, intuition will echo through your mind if you empty it.

In the stillness, the universe will guide your way.

Be the key that unlocks the Age of Awareness, the Age of Enlightenment.

Be the key, and turn the handle.

Sat Nam.

Now what?

*T*here's always more to learn, somewhere higher to go.

Let the God within you fan the flames, the passion for learning, and move ever higher with your soul.

Kundalini Yoga provides practical tools that anyone can apply in their life, tools that can awaken you to the God within if you apply them.

What higher purpose is there than awakening to the reality that you are God and doing God's work?

Well?

Walk in the stillness

*L*et your radiance shine through with a purity of thought and action.

Ray Man eh, Sat Nam.

Let the light of your truth be a beacon that shines in the night.

Open your heart to the song of your soul and be love.

Walk in the stillness that is an empty mind and be the angel of peace.

Free your mind and free your soul of all burden.

Meditate on the emptiness, meditate unto Infinity.

God's calling....

Sat Nam.

Between the footprints

*F*ollow in between the footprints and see where I've been.

Walk where I've walked if you choose.

I'm not the source of any of these teachings. I'm just the messenger, the guy with the bucket of water. Yogi Bhajan brought Kundalini Yoga to the West, and this book, it just comes to me and I write it down.

It's a very meditative circle. I relax and it flows through me, these descriptions of my experiences. Some things seem beyond words, as consciously pondering them brings nothing, empty the mind and it will flow through you.

It's brought me a much deeper understanding of so many things. It's what inspires me to push myself up off the floor one more time and then another, to get up hours before dawn and fold myself up into most restrictive posture imaginable and let go of every single thing that keeps me from being the lighthouse.

At first the pain was almost unbearable. It lessens with each passing day as I surrender to the posture. I can't imagine my life without it now, this Bound Lotus.

Find a meditation and yoga set that resonates with you. Share your experiences and inspire the world to be ten times greater than yourself.

Sat Nam.

Master the mind

*T*here's been times where I've nearly lost my mind, falling prey to the distractions, worrying instead of relaxing.

The hold those distractions have over you fades as the strength of your own personal practice, your sadhana increases.

Surrendering to fear or distractions is never an option. Yes, it takes work and it takes focus.

Meditation focuses and trains the mind, it can help break the hold those distractions have over your mind.

It's your mind, who's in charge, you or it?

Master the mind and walk with God.

Sat Nam.

The Infinite within

*D*on't simply exchange one distraction for another, unplug, relax and float in consciousness.

Hold truth in your heart and feel the Infinite within.

Doubt fades like light at sunset, faith blossoms in its place, springing forth like flowers opening their eyes for the very first time.

Let the fidgeting pass through you, look into your soul and see God.

To have come so far, keep going, keep on climbing that proverbial mountain of truth and discover God within.

Sat Nam.

Tomorrow

*B*ound Lotus, Day 123.

An angel sat down beside me this morning and wrapped its golden wings around me as I surrendered to the posture.

We chanted together, its soft feathers bringing divine relaxation.

Its bringing friends tomorrow....

Every day the experience deepens immeasurably, I wonder what tomorrow will be like....

Listen

*L*isten....

Become the silence and accept what comes to you.

Be that eagle of liberation and take flight into the vibration.

Let the sound waves wash over you and penetrate every cell of your being as you sink into oneness with the Infinite.

Wherever the ride takes you, enjoy it and vibrate with the Infinite.

Sat Nam.

Whispers on the wind

A trio of angels came to chant with me this morning.

They whispered into my mind, *"It's easy,"* and it was!

Wahe Guru!

Angels watch over you, always, invite them into your life and take them into your heart. Walk with them, look life in the eye and let go.

Sat Nam.

Heaven

*S*o what is Bound Lotus you ask?

It's not just a posture or a meditation, it's a call to God.

It's the sun, the moon, the stars and the entire universe in the palm of your hand. For me, it's heaven on Earth.

It's all that and so much more.

Do the work, carry the bucket of water, be the lighthouse and find your own slice of heaven on Earth.

Sat Nam.

Play consciously

*I*t all begins with a thought, a spark of creation from the universe.

Move through it, awake and aware.

Pause and be.

Listen, God's calling.

Wake up and move outside of the game once and for all.

We're all in this game called life, play consciously....

Grow with it

*L*ove crystallizes all around you as your vibration increases.

The path to consciousness is paved with love, open yourself to the experience.

Release the struggle and hear the angels singing you to sleep.

Allow the separation between you and the Infinite to evaporate, swim in consciousness, free....

Become the vibration, feel the energy within, growing with you as you become the lighthouse.

Sat Nam.

The wellspring of life

*T*he energy rises up through the stillness.

Become the posture and allow the mind, body and spirit to merge into consciousness.

Awaken the energy within and drink of the wellspring of life.

Transcend so called limits and rise up with the energy.

Walk in the stillness and take control of your life.

Now who wants to do some yoga, raise your hand.

Long time sun

*I*t all begins in the stillness, how you get there is entirely up to you.

Be, in the stillness, know and feel the universe vibrating through and all around you.

Relax, breathe, feel the energy rising within, transcend the self, move beyond pain, fear and doubt, wake up to the reality that you are divine and that the long time sun will truly shine upon you.

Sat Nam.

Escape the game

Go beyond time and space, focus on the silence and be in the now.

Float along on waves of consciousness as the barriers to awareness dissolve into nothingness.

Escape the game once and for all and be the lighthouse.

Sat Nam.

Where are you?

We will always be at the Ghost Ranch, my fellow Ghost Rancheros and I.

From now until the end of time, our words and deeds will hold the space they were created in.

Lanette's giant bonfires will burn for all eternity.

The stars will forever shine upon us, as the deer graze upon the alfalfa.

Yes my friends, we will always be at the Ghost Ranch, where we stood together and declared, "I am the lighthouse."

Sat Nam.

Children of God

We will always be, children of God, and things will always be just that, things.

Wrapped into the symbol for Infinity, there is no escape, only surrender. Who wins is up to you.

Surrender to the posture and let the healing begin. Surrender and see the sun rise and set at the same time, see yourself here, there, and back again all in the blink of an eye.

Let creativity flow, hear the whispers on the wind… God's calling.

Come what may, face it head on, chin held high.

Let Ong Namo Guru Dev Namo be thy sword and shield as you conquer the mind.

Sat Nam.

A game called life

Life is out here, not caught up in the game.

What game are you playing?

There is no reset button on this game called life, you can't just reboot and start back at the beginning, but you do have the power to change everything.

Swan dive into love, radiate from the heart, and discover life.

Getting there is up to you, it's all about the choices we make.

Where one journey ends, another begins.

What we create along the way is up to us.

What will you create?

Thought provoking questions? Tales from the road less traveled? A journey that never ends....

Drifting on the wind

Days spent drifting on the wind, nights riding on a comet....

That's what Bound Lotus is like.

The same three angels returned this morning, to share in the experience of surrender.

When we finished chanting they opened a window into their existence, what it is to be pure energy.

Then again, it's all just different views of the same experience....

Empty spaces

Now I understand why Yogi Bhajan taught to that empty classroom all those years ago.

Angels come to fill in the empty spaces.

The energy created will stay in that space for all time.

It's a reminder that as a teacher, you're not the source of the teachings, but rather a vehicle for them.

It's a direct experience of who and where you are.

It's a long deep look in the mirror and even an exercise in humility.

Try it sometime.

Sat Nam.

Sing with angels and touch the sun

*T*his is your invitation to sing with angels and touch the sun. Reach out and accept it....

Invest in yourself and invest in the future. Make peace your legacy and help create a world you would be proud to inherit.

Whether it ends in flame or light depends on what we as a race create. I've chosen the light....

Clear out those cobwebs and move from karma into dharma. Create consciously and be the lighthouse.

Sing with angels and touch the sun.

Sat Nam.

Choose it

*J*ust as all rivers end up in the ocean, all paths lead back to God.

Light that fuse and blast off, be the rocket ship of peace and light the way for the entire universe. Guide their way home.

Choose it and find inner peace in the blink of an eye. Choose it and watch the sun set on fourteen worlds. Choose it, smile and see God smile in the mirror.

Be the lighthouse, choose it, and be the lighthouse.

Sat Nam.

Where the ride takes you

*T*his started out at my first White Tantric Yoga, my first experience with anything of that magnitude. That day changed my life and that's where I wrote one of the earliest parts of this book. Of course, back then, I had no idea it would lead to a book, let alone everything that followed.

That's the beautiful thing about the path, go where it takes and grow along the way.

It comes to me and I write it down. A lot of it is guidance and not just for myself as I know this is meant to be shared. As my friend Catherine keeps reminding me, it's a gift from God, share it.

It just comes to me. At all different times, guiding my way home, helping me to relax, unplug and be in the present moment.

Some of it's even in the form of an open letter to my fellow Ghost Rancheros, my classmates from our Kundalini Yoga teacher training at the Ghost Ranch in New Mexico. My brothers and sisters….

We all changed high in the desert, reborn into lighthouses when we accepted our spiritual names, stood on the mountain and let go of the old, limited us that was that other person before we stood and declared, "I am the lighthouse!"

Pursue your passions and go where the ride takes you.

Sat Nam.

For everyone

*T*he writing and I evolve together, it literally just flows through me.

This is for everyone who loves to do frogs, for everyone who's ever chanted with me and for everyone who helped me to become the lighthouse. For all my friends, teachers and fellow lighthouses, bless you, thank you.

For Catherine, my number one fan, biggest supporter and endless supplier of inspirational talks. The Frisbee will always just miss you!

For Hari Ram, YOU are the lighthouse.

For Naomi, fellow Aries, explorer and mountain climber.

For Shabdh Singh, and his help with Sodarshan Chakra Kriya.

For Rebekah who helped us all to remember, "I am, I am."

For Har Hari and her unbridled enthusiasm. Wahe Guru!

For Sat Atma, her golden smile and amazing strength.

For Peggy and the rock she had us all sign so we would always be with her.

For Joel never giving up long after most would have.

For LaDawn and her angelic voice.

For Tim and his healing touch upon all our injuries.

For Zaloa hopping across the field on her crutches until her ankle healed.

For all the deer who come to hear us chant, and for the stars that shined down upon us as we all healed.

For Lanette and her bonfires that will always burn high into the night sky.

For Guru Meher who pushed until we knew we had no limits.

For Devi Dyal Singh and all the wisdom he so graciously imparted.

For Dr. Siri Atma and Nam Kaur sharing themselves with us.

For Scarlett who made me feel like a kid again.

For Devi Dyal Kaur who trusted me to operate on her foot.

For Satpal who finished her teacher training despite having to leave to go to the hospital.

For Hari and Ravi who made all of this happen. A monumental undertaking if ever there was one! Wahe Guru!

For Jenny and one sentence that touched me like never before, thank you.

For everyone I've ever met and who has helped me on my way home, this exists because of you.

For Lynn and China and all of their smiles and energy.

For Dev Suroop and Sangeet Kaur who taught us how to chant.

For Audur and the ladies of my triangle pose crew, I practice every day!

For Zoe who always pushed herself, stretching just to that point where she could barely hold it.

For David looking after me doing all my hiking and telling me I was as quiet as a ninja.

For Bruce and three of the funniest words I've ever heard, "Sat Nam eh."

For Taina who traveled halfway around the world to become the lighthouse and to become a teacher in a land without one.

For Gurmit, Patrice and Bonita who made similar incredibly long journeys to be the lighthouse.

For all of our family who came from far away, traveling all the way across this country or from another one.

For Sergio, one of the quietest and yet most fascinating and wisest people I've ever met.

For Erin and Rosario, neighbors who were always there to listen and offer support.

For John, another neighbor and fellow writer, may you always live in a moment of Wahe Guru!

For Merritt, always looking after her dad, when he couldn't.

For Joe who left the old Joe behind to become Sat Daya.

For Heidi, my neighbor with a smile and laundry detergent for everyone.

For Agnieszka whose smiles and energy brightened all our lives.

For Jiwan Shakti who came all the way across the country to cut watermelon with me and help us all to be the lighthouse.

For Christine and her happy go dancing with her MP3 player ways.

For Jennifer who also left her job to be the lighthouse.

For Karma, whose family brought us all a little touch of home.

For Maura who left her home in the mountains to become a lighthouse.

For Christy who somehow kept up during White Tantric Yoga on almost no sleep.

For all my hiking companions and the eagle that watched over us.

For those like Anastasia and Priti Kaur who also came from far away or Nirbhao, Sat Jiwan and Andrea who journeyed cross country, or DeDee and Pat who had shorter journeys yet still left so much behind so they could help others. No matter how far we physically traveled, everyone made a journey of sorts and left something behind, to be the lighthouse.

For everyone who ever said Sat Nam or Ong Namo.

For Sat Hari who led the way up the mountain and showed me the true nature of strength.

For Chris, who had never even done yoga, but went to Winter Solstice because his sister asked him to as her Christmas present.

For my parents.

For my Bound Lotus mentor, Sat Nam Kaur and the greatest gift ever, Wahe Guru!

For Guru Gobind Singh who has blessed me with his energy and support.

And for Yogi Bhajan who made all of this possible.

Sat Nam.

Wherever you are on your path, acknowledge it, how you got there and all those who helped you along the way. Let creativity flow through you, become that empty vessel to be filled with truth and be the lighthouse, for everyone.

Sat Nam.

Get out of your own way

*B*ound Lotus, Day 134.

The first day it took everything I had to hold the posture for all of 30 seconds. I daresay 31 minutes is comfortable and even relaxing now.

Like anything else you work up to it. You don't start out to climb Mount Everest without having climbed something smaller first.

We all have to start somewhere and I most certainly did not start out writing about yoga and being a lighthouse. But along the way it grew into something far larger than myself as I got out of my own way.

It gives me the chills to think that it's evolved to where it inspires people. That's pretty profound… I'm just the guy with the bucket of water.

Get out of your own way and let it flow through you.

Focus on the stillness and the energy rises, focus on the distractions and it sinks, it's as simple as that.

So come on, sit down and we'll do some yoga together.

The games we play

We spend our entire lives playing one game or another.

What game are you playing?

There are many games within the game of life. Some help you along the path while others pull you from it.

What game could possibly be more fun than emptying that proverbial garbage pit and freeing your mind?

What could bring greater peace than stilling the mind and feeling the kundalini rising?

Well?

Clear out those chakras and blow out the cobwebs.

It's your garbage pit, you can keep filling it up or you can empty it out....

Sat Nam.

Who's with me?

What will you commit to?

Right now, will you stand with me and declare, "I am the lighthouse?"

What commitment will you make towards freeing your mind?

There is no silence in the stillness, only energy and the layers of vibration.

Discern the separate sounds and feel them echo throughout the entirety of your being.

Ultimately the mind and soul stand naked before the Infinite, clothed only in energy and vibration.

Make them your constant companions and be the lighthouse.

Sat Nam.

Walk with me

*T*rust in yourself and go where the path takes you, be it up or down.

Ride the waves to freedom and liberation.

Let go and be.

It's not about the money and understanding will come through the stillness.

Seek them not, they will find you through the stillness.

Walk with me, into the light.

Sat Nam.

How far you get

*P*eace comes through stillness, not chasing about.

Detachment not attachment.

Feel the dawn approaching and rise up with it.

Whether you set out to climb Mount Everest, do a thousand frogs, or take out the garbage, do it with a smile and give it your best effort.

How far you get doesn't matter nearly as much as what you put into it.

Sat Nam.

Be your own inspiration

What comes through the stillness is up to you.

Listen and be.

Challenge yourself beyond imagination and prove once and for all that the only limits are the ones we place upon ourselves.

There'll be days where achieving even 30 percent of your goal will be a tremendous success.

See it not as a failure but for the triumph it truly is and be your own inspiration.

Sat Nam.

See the wind

The vibration becomes clearer as you give yourself to it.

Blood soaked fields afar, "No more," cries the wind.

No one listens, no one's left… they've all gone….

"Where," cries the wind, but the watchmen are gone, long since turned to ash….

"Here," sound the watchmen turned angels, "look up."

It's your path, no one can walk it for you, and where it goes is up to you. Give yourself to the vibration and see all around you. See the wind itself, fly with angels and be the lighthouse.

Sat Nam.

Where the path takes you

*V*ibrate until the body no longer exists.

Open your awareness and reach out in all directions with every sense.

Ascend to new heights with every realization and let the sharks fight over their scraps of meat.

Give yourself to the vibration and leave them to their games.

Let go, and in that instant, have everything you've ever wanted but couldn't have. Then again, you won't want it anymore… quite the interesting conundrum isn't it?

Go where the path takes you and see it through.

Believe in yourself and the rest will take care of itself.

Sat Nam.

Reactions

I think, for me, the most special thing about all of this is the reactions I get from it.

It's profound, to invoke such deep, heartfelt responses, and I share in the laughter too….

I'm just a guy, the guy with the bucket of water, and when I say it just comes to me, it literally just does, and I write it down.

Bless you, Sat Nam.

The day will come

*T*he day will come, when you'll have the answers before you ever even have the question.

The day will come, when you quit asking questions and become the answers.

When you quit chasing happiness and let go, and let the light shine through.

The day will come, when you'll experience neither want nor need.

The day will come, when you will be, and walk in the light.

Until that day comes, keep on climbing that proverbial mountain of truth and be the lighthouse.

Sat Nam.

Proof positive

*T*here's a certain magic about coming from the Ghost Ranch, maybe it's something in the air there.

Then again, maybe it's the experiences we all shared there, being shaped into lighthouses and all.

I know for me, the three weeks I spent there are proof positive that the light will always shine and brightly at that.

Sat Nam.

I'll be there

When you need me, speak my name and I'll be there.

Whether a whisper in the wind or but a thought, the light is always with you, as is God.

I am there, before you even have the thought, I am everywhere for I am God and so are you.

Sat Nam.

You will always be

Times come, when you don't want to see into the future….

Sooner or later we are all confronted with our own immortality.

Our mortality does in part define who you are but the soul carries the experiences of all our lifetimes into eternity.

The desire to escape into the game grows strong if allowed. Face reality and be the game. It's your game, it's your rules, and you can play any way you choose. You can change the game at any time and you can always choose to play a higher game.

But no matter how you play, see it for the game that it is. Life is eternal. It's easy to become caught up in the physical and lose sight of that.

You will always be.

Sat Nam.

Pinkish haze

*T*he greatest adventure ever, the one my writing has taken me on. We grow together….

The energy pulses like waves upon the shore.

Pinkish haze as the sun bids good eve to this land, energy on the rise.

Whatever the noise, the vibration is always there… listen….

Your light will be too bright for some, shine on.

Some will doubt your words, as it is not to their purpose, shine on.

Shine on in the face of adversity and everything else the universe throws at you. Shine on and be the lighthouse.

Sat Nam.

Still others

*S*till others will doubt the words of the greatest masters to ever have walked this planet simply because they wish to do otherwise.

If they cling to their beliefs, that's their choice. Believe in the light, believe in yourself, feel and know that you are God.

May the light ever guide your way on.

Sat Nam.

Golden city on the water

*G*olden city on the water....

Where they live and breathe Ong Namo....

City of light, truth and peace....

I'd like to teach the world those five little words, their meaning and importance....

Ong Namo Guru Dev Namo....

Until that day, carry the water and be the lighthouse.

Sat Nam.

Stairway to heaven

*S*it and be with the energy.

Let it climb that magical staircase through the spine, let it tingle through the brain and pour out into the aura as you relax into the stillness.

Sit and be.

Master the moment and live in the now.

Be at peace, be at rest and be the lighthouse.

Sit without effort, tall, chin in, chest out.

Dwell in the stillness and let the energy flow....

Sat Nam.

Home

*I*s home where your yoga mat is, or is it a place filled with things?

How we define the world around us helps define who and what we are as a person.

Sit, meditate and the energy will come.

Will you work for it? Will you wait for it?

Rise up with the energy and taste the sunshine. Touch the unlimited potential within, walk with angels and be the lighthouse.

Sat Nam.

Leap of faith

*J*ust as every path has its own set of distractions, so too does each path have its own chasm, a cliff or canyon of some sort, crossable only by a leap of faith.

Decide you must, whether to abandon the path entirely or to make that leap, trusting in yourself and in the universe, knowing your success is guaranteed.

Be the eagle of liberation and leave the nest and all of its distractions far behind. Let go of the path, take that plunge into the light and awaken to consciousness.

No one can make that leap for you and the decision is yours....

What will you do?

Tune in and find out.

"Ong Namo Guru Dev Namo."

Let go, leave behind that which no longer serves you and let's all get to that golden city on the water. It's there waiting for us….

Sat Nam.

A breathless breath

I exist in my own universe now, outside of space and time, from the city on the water in the land of Ong Namo, and you can too.

You don't have to play the games or be caught up in the machinations of the world around you. It just is, what are you?

Are you the answer or are you the question?

I had no idea where this was leading when I started out, yet I did it anyway, and you can too.

Breathe a breathless breath, be in the stillness and let the energy flow.

Sat Nam.

Distractions

T he game calls, offering exhilaration and entertainment, but at what price?

Yes the game is fun, but what does it keep you from doing?

Your sadhana?

Being the lighthouse?

Writing this book?

What is it about the game that makes it so enticing?

Yes of course it's fun, but what does the game have to do with freeing your mind and serving others?

It's a distraction plain and simple.

Let's do something constructive instead. Now who's up for some yoga? Raise your hand.

In the game

*K*nock knock.

Are you here or are you in the game?

Shuniya, breathless, no movement, zero.

When you become nothing, that's when the energy comes.

I find myself in the game all too often, as if it exerts some otherworldly influence on me….

It's a choice though, we always have choice.

Play every game with detachment, even life, after all, it's all just a game.

Watch yourself breathe and be the game.

Watch the energy rise and be in the moment.

Sat Nam.

The journey through Ong Namo

Will you make the journey with me?

The journey through Ong Namo?

To be the lighthouse through the long dark to uphold light and truth in all that you do?

To shine on in the face of seemingly overwhelming adversity?

Let's make the journey together.

Sat Nam.

Change

The world around you changes along with you.

Things you once deemed to be of great importance will seem trivial.

Worry gets left by the side of the road, right next to desire and attachment.

Eventually even the ego will end up by the side of the road.

So, why would anyone not do their yoga?

Well?

Know yourself

*K*now yourself and know God.

Knowing the path is fine and even fun sometimes, but you still have to walk down it, no matter where it leads….

Some days you don't want to….

The light shines for everyone, will you drink of it?

The lighthouse doesn't see its own light, it shines for everyone else.

It shines so others can find their way home.

Follow the path back to the light and be the lighthouse.

Sat Nam.

Doei Shabd Kriya

*A*nd then we come to the miracle of creation that is Doei Shabd Kriya.

God's doorstep….

Sat Nam Wahe Guru.

Even just three minutes is a direct call to the energy within, the kundalini, and does it ever answer!

You call it, it rises, it's as simple as that.

Call on the energy and experience your divinity, it's your birthright.

Sat Nam.

God's doorstep

*D*oei Shabd Kriya delivers you to God's doorstep. Do the work and that door will open into your mind.

Sat Nam Wahe Guru.

Take that journey into the center of your mind and watch as the entire universe seemingly spins around you.

See into the black vastness of the universe, out through your own mind, touch your own divinity, know that you are infinite and that we are all children of God.

No limits, not now, not ever.

Sat Nam

Pick one

I would have thought, that seeing as how awesome Doei Shabd Kriya is, there'd be all kinds of stuff written about it, all over the place. Yet all that exists is a single page in a single book… until now that is!

Therein lies the magic that is Kundalini Yoga.

There are literally hundreds and hundreds of amazingly powerful kriyas and meditations with Kundalini Yoga.

Pick one or two, or ten, make them your own, perfect them, and be the lighthouse.

Sat Nam.

To carry you through the night

Given the tremendous power of words, how much attention do we pay to the words we use?

A single sentence can be the mightiest of swords that inspires one in the darkest of hours.

A lighthouse gives you that sentence to carry with you, now and for all time, for when the going gets rough.

Thank you Nam for giving me that one sentence.

Sat Nam.

Let it echo

Let the sound of Ong Namo Guru Dev Namo echo throughout the land and the light shall pour forth from the golden city on the water.

Feel the Ray Man Shabad live and breath as you surrender to the posture.

Let the hills come alive with the sound of Ek Ong Kar, Sat Nam and Wahe Guru.

Dance with Hari Har, touch the sky and rejoice unto the light.

May Aud Guray Nameh stand between you and harm in all the dark places you must walk.

With Saa Re Saa Saa as your armor and Ong Namo as your sword and shield no darkness shall ever defeat thee.

Stand tall and radiate unto the Infinite. Shine on through the days and nights, be the lighthouse and guide everyone home.

Sat Nam.

Echoes in the mist

*F*ascinating, the myriad lines of confluence that come together to create the events of our lives.

For instance, I quit my job to become a yoga teacher. Along the way I also became a writer and a web designer. Yes, I still teach, but who would have thought the one would have led to the others?

Then again, yoga and my writing are inextricably linked, growing in unison as I continue down the path….

Where does it all lead?

Where does your path lead?

If you knew, would you still walk down it?

Let's get there together, maybe there's a rainbow….

Sat Nam.

Answer the call

*T*here's something about the unparalleled majesty of an eagle in flight that immediately draws ones attention skyward.

Their unmistakable call grabs you like some great unseen hand calling you to the sky.

Your soul's calling you down the path, answer the call and be the lighthouse.

Sat Nam.

Trust in Nanak

I have a very dear friend, I always marvel at how she can say a million things with but one short sentence.

To be able to provoke such thought and instill such inspiration one with just three words....

Wahe Guru!

Even a lighthouse needs inspiration at times, when it gets dark and you fall....

A great hand will always reach out and catch you. Trust in Nanak, trust in yourself, and trust in the universe, your success is already guaranteed, all you have to do is achieve it.

Sat Nam.

Three miles up, three miles down

*H*ow far would you travel on a friend's invitation?

To see them smile, to brighten their day, because they asked you to….

How far will you carry the bucket of water?

How far will you carry the light?

In the end, when the question is, "Did I uplift enough?" what will your answer be?

Don't leave doubt when you know you can do more.

Touch everyone you meet, make every encounter meaningful, even if all you can do is bring a smile to their face.

Uplift everyone you meet and be the lighthouse.

Sat Nam.

Why not?

*W*ings beneath my feet, nothing but the blue and the white as far as the eye can see.

Almost as if the clouds were a mighty soup one could reach out and scoop up….

Timeless, ageless, thoughtless, motionless motion, moving without moving, high above the all, living in the vibration….

The faster you hurry the slower you go, so why hurry?

Why not smell the fresh air and taste freedom like never before?

Why not touch the sky and soar with eagles?

Why not?

Why not free your mind?

Why not?

In my mother's arms

*A*s safe as when I was in my mother's arms.

I knew no harm would come to me, cradled in God's arms, when the light was all there was.

Before the darkness came and the reality of the modern world thrust itself upon the sanctity of my parents' creation—me—the guy with the bucket of water.

Come, drink if you wish.

Sat Nam.

Stop and listen

*T*he masses scurry about the big city, chasing time.

Perpetually late, they hurry to make up for "lost" time.

How pray tell do you lose time?

Not even in their hustling can they escape the vibration.

Too busy to hear it, they continue to chase that which they cannot lose. It's the chasing about that keeps them from their goal.

Stop and listen....

Turn the key

*O*ng Namo is the key to the ultimate journey.

That's where it all begins....

Turn the key and take the road less traveled.

Journey with me, into the unknown, to a sacred realm beyond space and time.

One where Sat Nam, Wahe Guru and the vibration live and breathe.

A land where the light takes form and angels dance....

Take control of your mind and turn the key.

Sat Nam.

Angel's playground

*S*hells crunch beneath the feet, crystal clear water to Infinity... footsteps along the path....

At long last, the top of the mountain, a lighthouse led the way....

Trees that reach to the heavens, where the emerald green water flows... footsteps through the angel's playground... the land of Ong Namo....

Keep on climbing and find that golden city on the water, no matter where it is for you.

Sat Nam.

The land of Ong Namo

At long last, the golden city on the water, where the air itself is alive with the sound of Ong Namo Guru Dev Namo....

At last, I've found the land of Ong Namo! Wahe Guru!

It lies within my heart, for it isn't a physical place one can reach by any ordinary means.

But rather it's a state of mind, a choice, a lifestyle if you will, a decision, to stand tall against the darkness no matter the consequences, to uphold light and truth in all that you do and be the lighthouse.

Sat Nam.

For Bruce

"A thousand blessings my friend," the man in black said, and blessed I am!

I've been everywhere man, I've been to Phoenix, Sante Fe, Albuquerque, Abiquiu, Espanola, Ocala, Chicago, Denver, St. Louis, Ottawa, Toronto, Vancouver, Sydney, Perth, Los Angeles, Peoria, Dayton, Gettysburg, Miami, Winter Solstice, Summer Solstice, I've been everywhere man!

And I've even been to the one place you can't reach by trying to get there—the golden city on the water in the land of Ong Namo.

I've been everywhere man, carried on the wings of my many blessings.

Wherever you are on your journey, be thankful for each and every one of your blessings. May they be many.

Sat Nam.

Footsteps in the mist

Yet another journey, yet another bald eagle….

There is hope for us, for we've brought the most majestic of creatures back from the brink of extinction.

Now if only we could flourish like the eagles have….

I wonder what the eagles would teach us if they could, if only we could understand them… perhaps we could soar, live and be free… free of pain and suffering….

It'll happen, if we all find the land of Ong Namo, where there are no cell phones, computers, or even televisions....

Make that journey to the land of Ong Namo and be the lighthouse.

Sat Nam.

And so it begins

*T*he book might come to an end, but the journey never will. This is only the beginning....

Yes, I've glimpsed what lies ahead, but I still have to walk down that road, just as you must walk down yours. Come, let's get there together.

That being said, bless you and thank you one and all. May the long time sun ever shine its loving light upon you and of course, be the lighthouse!

Thank you Guru Gobind Singh for all of your energy and support.

Thank you Yogi Bhajan for your courage, vision, strength and for bringing Kundalini Yoga to the West.

And thank you God for ever being my friend and for making all of this possible.

Thank you God for every bump on my knee, every ecstasy, every pain and every joy I've ever had or ever will have.

Thank you God for helping me to be the lighthouse and for helping me to carry the bucket of water.

Thank you God for every thing, bless you.

Sat Nam.

Resources

*F*or more information on Bound Lotus, please visit Mahan Kirn Kaur Khalsa's website at www.boundlotus.com

To find a KRI Certified Instructor near you, please visit the International Kundalini Yoga Teachers Association (IKYTA) website at www.kundaliniyoga.com.

For more information on Kundalini Yoga Events visit www.3ho.org

For Kundalini Yoga products and Yogi Bhajan DVDs visit www.a-healing.com

Printed in the United States
64965LVS00006B/1-150

9 781598 581881